robert jones'

makeup
masterclass

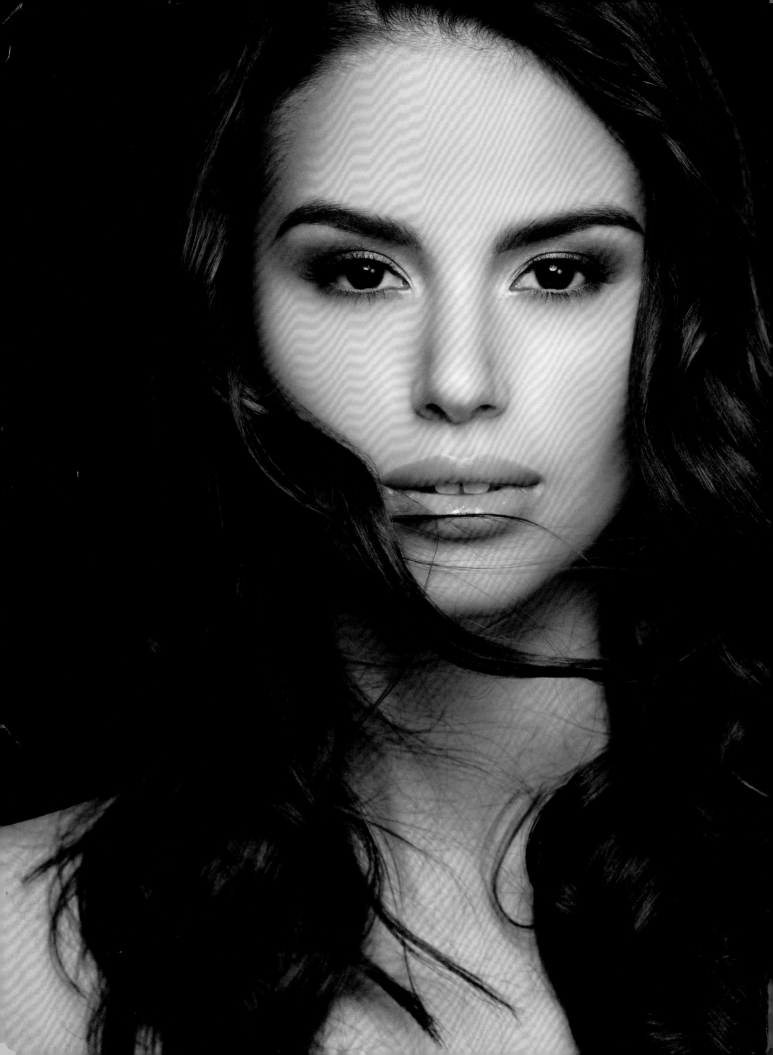

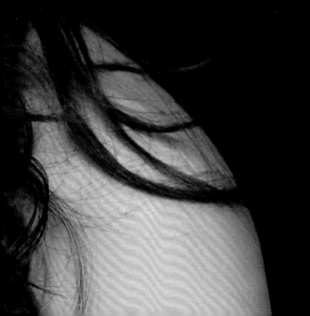

robert jones'
makeup
masterclass

a complete course in
makeup for all levels, beginner to advanced

robert jones, international makeup artist, robertjonesbeauty.com

FAIR WINDS

acknowledgments

I need to thank Greg Stephens, Tim Stewart, and Linda Sambera. Without these three people, this book would never have happened. Your amount of work and dedication was immeasurable and invaluable. It only exists because of you three.

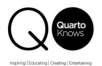

Brimming with creative inspiration, how-to projects, and useful information to enrich your everyday life, Quarto Knows is a favorite destination for those pursuing their interests and passions. Visit our site and dig deeper with our books into your area of interest: Quarto Creates, Quarto Cooks, Quarto Homes, Quarto Lives, Quarto Drives, Quarto Explores, Quarto Gifts, or Quarto Kids.

ISBN: 978-1-59233-783-5

Digital edition published in 2018

Library of Congress Cataloging-in-Publication Data available.

Design and page layout: Sporto

hair and makeup: robert jones, www.robertjonesbeauty.com
representation: seaminx artist management, www.seaminx.com
photography: greg stephens, www.gregstephens.com
photo assistant: tim stewart, www.timstewartphoto.com
still-life photography: fernando ceja, www.fernandoceja.com
still-life styling: phillip groves, www.onsetmanagement.com
illustrations: finis jordan, www.finisjordan.com

© 2018 Quarto Publishing Group USA Inc.
Text © 2018 Robert Jones

First Published in 2018 by Fair Winds Press, an imprint of The Quarto Group, 100 Cummings Center, Suite 265-D, Beverly, MA 01915, USA.
T (978) 282-9590 F (978) 283-2742
QuartoKnows.com

Fair Winds Press titles are also available at discount for retail, wholesale, promotional, and bulk purchase. For details, contact the Special Sales Manager by email at specialsales@quarto.com or by mail at The Quarto Group, Attn: Special Sales Manager, 401 Second Avenue North, Suite 310, Minneapolis, MN 55401, USA.

21 20 19 18 17   1 2 3 4 5

dedication

This book is dedicated to all the future makeup
artists of the world . . . but especially those who
pick up a makeup brush with the hope or
intention of making themselves or someone else
feel more confident and beautiful!

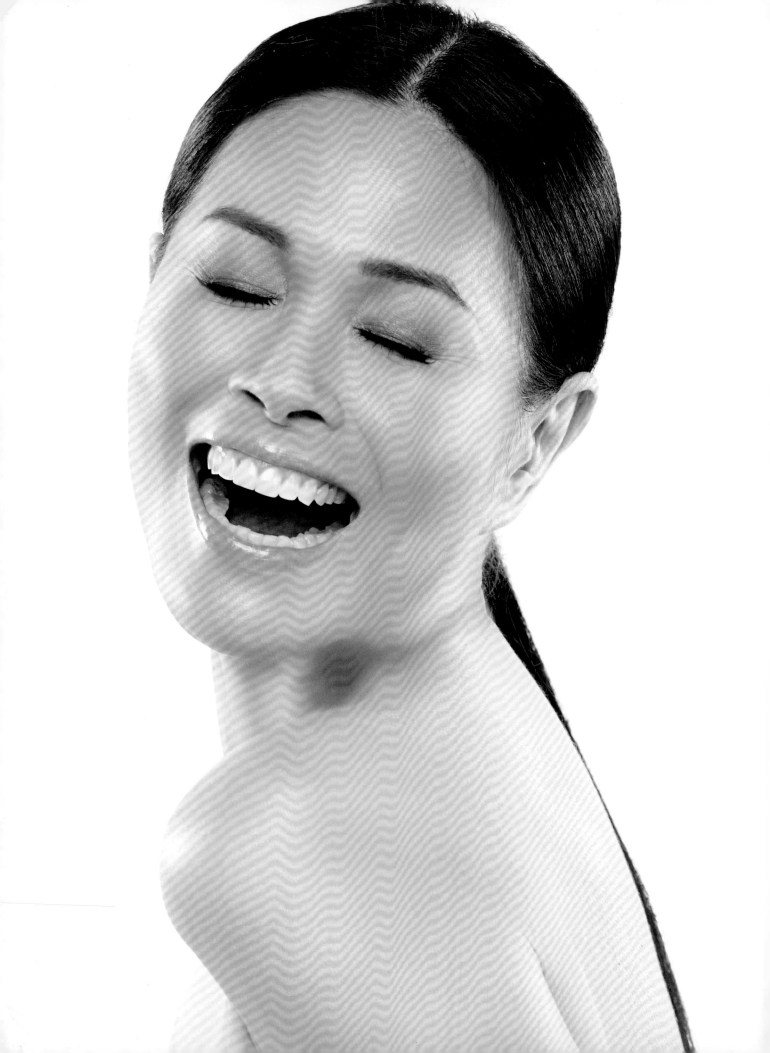

contents

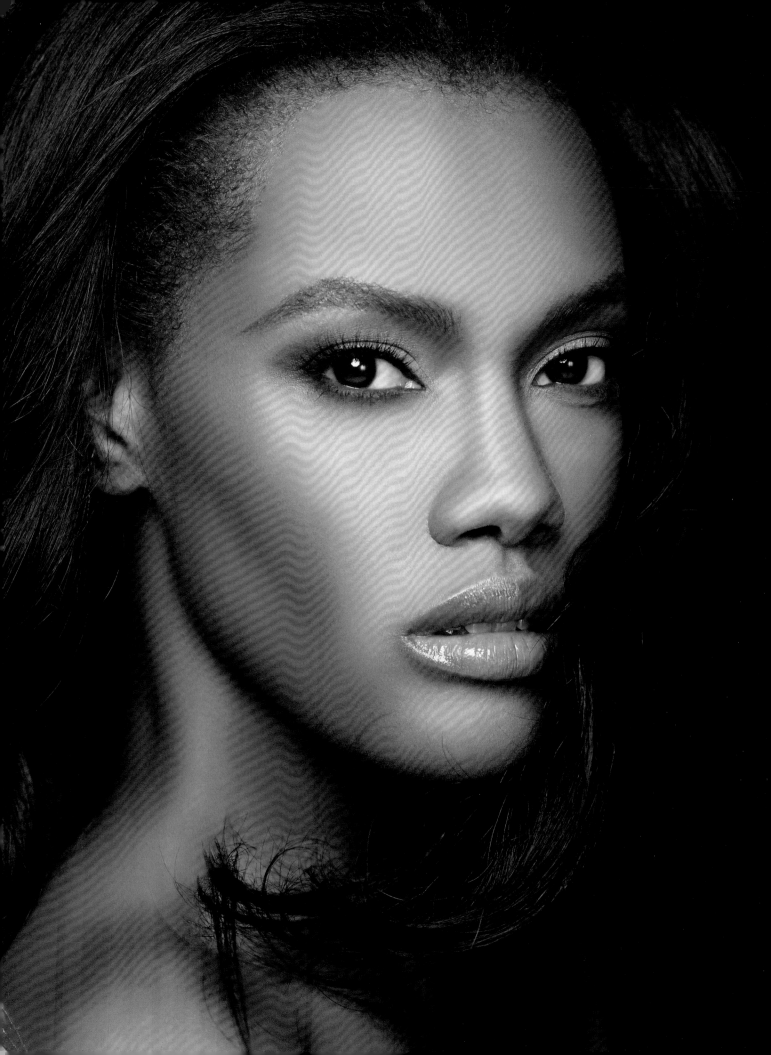

introduction

It's an age-old question: what is true beauty?

The answer is self-confidence, of course!

Self-confidence can immediately make someone look and feel more beautiful. And that's the real power of makeup: it can give you self-confidence like nothing else. I love being able to make such a big change with nothing more than a little makeup and some brushes. When you make someone feel beautiful on the outside, it is amazing what it does for them on the inside.

In this book, I'll give you all the information you need to reach your most confident self via makeup. Throughout my career, I've been amazed to watch what a difference feeling beautiful can make. I want to equip you with the tools you need to experience it as well.

Of course, there's an overwhelming amount of information about makeup out there, so it's hard to know where to start. My goal is to make it simple because it is!

I've broken it down to the absolute basics. No matter your skin tone or skin type, the information is here. Whether you are a beginner or someone with makeup experience, there is something here for you. And everything is laid out in a step-by-step way, so you can learn to be your own makeup artist.

We'll discuss all the tools and products that are out there, so you can make the best choices for yourself. After all, there isn't just one generic eye shadow application, for example, that works for everyone. You'll learn techniques to enhance every different eye shape and every different face shape. I'll explain how to accentuate—or hide—anything you might want to, so you can feel the best about your skin.

Then we will move on to explore how to combine these basic techniques to create more advanced looks. This is a makeup masterclass because when you are finished, you will not only have enough knowledge to do your own makeup, but you will have enough knowledge to do others' as well. Not only can you bring out your own self-confidence, you can help others bring out theirs too.

So let's get started exploring the world of makeup!

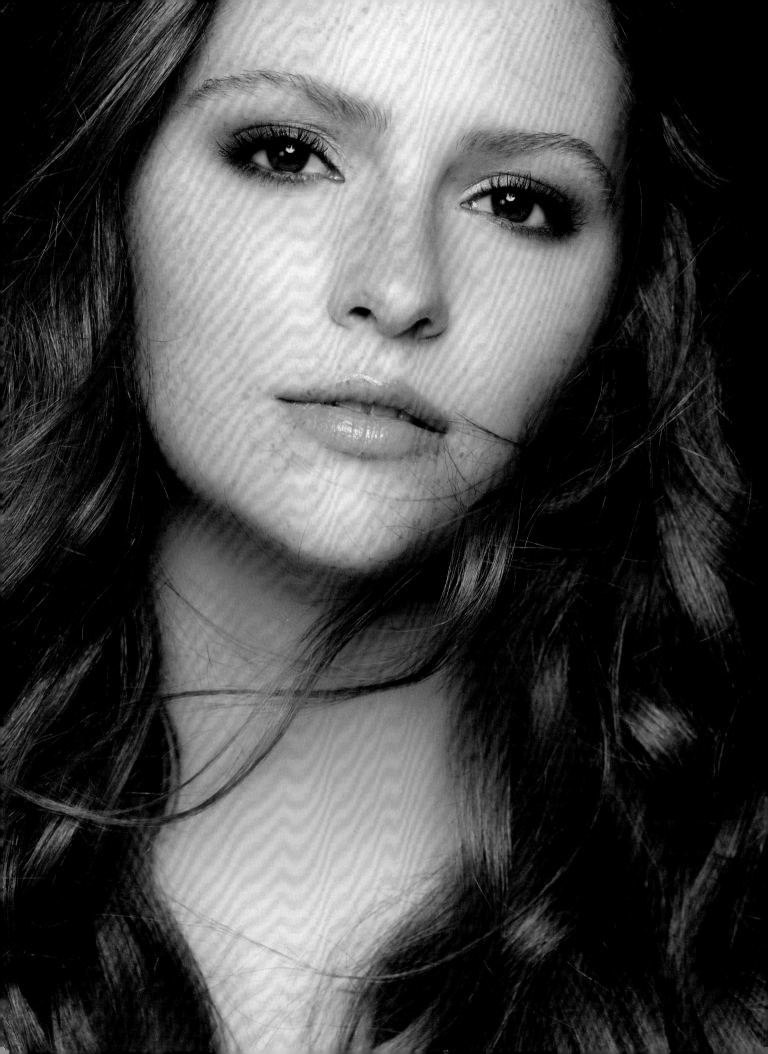

tools of the trade

One of the most confusing things about makeup is figuring out which products to choose. It's hard to know what to buy, where to invest the bulk of your money, and where to maybe save a dollar or two. There are so many questions: Which formula of foundation would work best for you? Which type of blush will be the easiest to apply? Which type of eyeliner will meet your needs? Do you want to wear lipstick or lip gloss?

If you go to a department store, you'll be hit with an endless number of products that the salesperson just wants to sell you. Many you do not need and probably will never wear. If you go to a drug store, there will be no one to help you, and you may not know what to do. Which is better?

The best solution is to educate yourself so you can make your best choices no matter where you are. In this chapter, we will discuss which products will best meet all your needs.

foundation

Foundation is the most important piece of makeup you will ever purchase. It can make your skin appear flawless and natural, with a healthy glow. It can cover imperfections and blemishes and smooth out uneven skin tones. The right one looks like you're wearing nothing; the wrong one looks like you're wearing a mask. The right one can erase years; the wrong one can add years. Wearing foundation correctly can do more for your appearance than practically any other makeup product. It can also be one of the most difficult to choose correctly.

When making your foundation choice, there are two things to consider. First, match your skin tone and depth so your foundation looks natural. Second, match your skin type with the correct foundation formula. For example, if you have oily skin, the oils can mix with the product and make your skin appear blotchy and uneven, so you need a foundation with oil absorbers in it. If you have dry skin, you need a foundation with moisturizers in it so it helps your skin look supple and fresh and keeps it from looking blotchy. Wearing the correct foundation formula for your skin type can help your foundation stay on longer and your skin look even and flawless.

My advice? Treat yourself to the best foundation you can afford. Higher priced foundations usually contain higher quality pigments that last longer and appear much more flattering. They also usually contain higher quality moisturizers and oil absorbers, helping them perform better. Cheaper foundations contain fewer, inferior pigments that usually don't wear as long.

Your skin is the most important part of your makeup look, and making it look the freshest and most flawless is so important. Foundation and powder are the bases of flawless-looking skin, so you should try to buy the best.

You have a lot of options when it comes to foundation formulations. Thanks to modern technology, many foundations can appear almost invisible. There are all kinds of new light-reflecting ingredients in foundation that will hide your flaws without piling on lots of product. There are all kinds of new pigment technologies making it an almost pure pigment that adds straight coverage with no weight or texture. If you want more coverage from your foundation, choose one with more pigment in it rather than using more of the product. Choose from a variety of textures and formulas that will give you different coverages and finishes. A product's consistency and the way it goes onto the skin is the key to even, flawless coverage.

The real goal is for your foundation to look as if you're not wearing any at all. You simply give the illusion of having healthy, glowing, flawless skin. Your skin changes with the seasons and as you age, and you must change your foundation as well if you want to continue looking flawless and fresh.

liquid foundation. This is the most popular foundation and is suited to most—if not all—skin types. It is available in every type of formula, from oil-free, oil-absorbing for oily skin to moisturizing for dry skin. Liquid foundation gives varying degrees of sheer to medium coverage, depending on the brand and the formula, so you can choose the amount of coverage you want. Most can be layered to create more coverage. You can purchase it in a bottle or a tube. It gives you more coverage than a tinted moisturizer, but less than a crème or stick foundation.

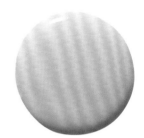

liquid pigment. This liquid foundation is almost pure pigment, giving you great coverage without weight and texture. It can be used alone or added to other products such as moisturizers, primers, tinted moisturizers, bb creams, or other foundations. The more drops you use, the more coverage you get; you completely control the coverage. It's great for all skin types, and it's one of my favorite formulas for coverage and natural appearance.

crème foundation. Smooth and creamy, crème foundation is specifically formulated for normal to very dry complexions. It's one of the most moisturizing formulas you can use. It gives the skin a natural finish while offering one of the highest of all coverages. It's also versatile—even though it tends to have a thicker and heavier consistency, it can be made sheerer if you apply it with a damp sponge (which also allows you to control the coverage). Crème foundation is great for dry skin. However, if you have flaky skin, it can look cakey, and the result can be slightly dull and heavy-looking.

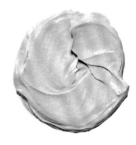

mousse foundation. This is a crème foundation that has a whipped consistency. Mousse foundations are formulated for normal to dry skin. Mousse generally comes in a jar rather than a compact, and it is usually lighter and sheerer than its compact counterpart. It evens out the skin tone without appearing heavy. Usually high in pigment and low in viscosity, it gives you great coverage while appearing almost invisible on the skin. I use mousse-textured formulas a lot because they seem to sink into the skin rather than sit on top of it. They give great coverage that appears very natural. They are fabulous on mature skin because they do not collect in fine lines like heavier crème formulas.

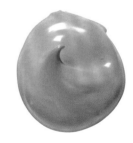

stick foundation. Stick foundation is essentially a neatly packaged crème foundation and concealer in one. Best for normal to dry skin, it is a good option if you want more coverage. It offers ideal maximum coverage for imperfections, as well as covering ruddy and uneven skin tones. Stick foundation will give you quick coverage, but it can look a little heavy on clear skin, on which a lot of coverage is not needed. The beauty of this formula is that you can dot it where you need it rather than applying it to your entire face. Then you can simply blend powder in and go.

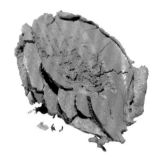

crème-to-powder foundation. This is quick and simple! Formulated for normal to slightly oily skin, it has a creamy texture that dries to a powder finish; usually no additional dusting of powder is needed to set it. These formulas are kinder to oily skin than their crème counterparts because the powder helps cut down on excess shine. Once again, because it is a crème at heart, it will give you more coverage. It offers a little less coverage than its moisturizing crème counterparts (crème and stick), but more than a liquid or tinted moisturizer.

bb, cc, and dd creams. These are lightweight, low coverage versions of a foundation with lots of treatment. We started with bb (beauty balm) creams, which were designed to brighten and lighten the skin while moisturizing and providing sunscreen. Then we got cc (color corrector or coverage control) creams with light but better coverage and built-in primer, brightener, and anti-aging properties. Some boast as many as twelve functions in one product. Now dd (daily defense or dermatologically defining) creams provide additional long-term anti-aging benefits with the increased coverage that we got added from our cc cream. I'm sure the alphabet will continue on as innovations in science and beauty emerge.

tinted moisturizer. This is moisturizer with a little color added. This formula works best on normal to dry skin and gives you sheer, lightweight, breathable coverage with a fresh, nearly naked finish. It gives you the sheerest coverage of all the foundation formulas, and it's ideal for use during the summer months when you feel like wearing next to nothing. It evens out your skin tone and is the easiest to apply due to its sheerness. Many brands contain sunscreen, which means one less step in the morning.

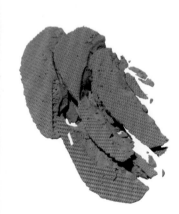

powder compact. This dual-finish powder foundation gives a quick and convenient sheer-to-medium coverage and is packaged in a nice neat compact. It is formulated for normal to oily skin; on dry skin, it will just look chalky. It goes on like a pressed powder but gives you slightly more coverage, because it contains emollients and pigments. It's a great choice for young girls because it is low in oils and moisturizers, so it does not clog pores, cutting down on the risk of breakouts. Also, it is all the coverage that most young girls need and is easy for them to apply. You control the coverage by choosing your tool of application. Applied with a brush, it gives you sheer coverage. Applied with a sponge, it gives you more complete coverage.

pigmented mineral powder. Loose powder that adheres to the skin, pigmented mineral powder provides sheer to medium coverage. It is formulated for normal to oily skin; on dry skin, it will appear too chalky. In addition to giving you coverage, it also contains vitamins and minerals, which make it great for sensitive skin. It works much like a dual-finish powder foundation and is simple to apply with a brush or a sponge. Applied with a brush, it gives you sheer to medium coverage. Applied

tip: *If your skin tends to flake, make sure you exfoliate to get rid of that top layer of dead, dry skin before applying a crème foundation.*

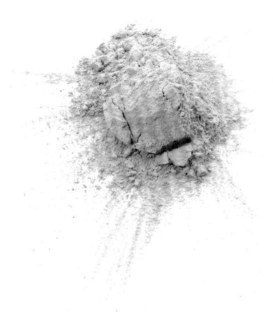

with a sponge, it gives you medium coverage (and if you apply enough layers, full coverage). With any tool, the more layers you apply, the more coverage you will get. Be careful, though: too much of this formula can look cakey, due to its powder consistency. It usually does not contain any preservatives, and like tinted moisturizer, it may also provide sunscreen.

airbrush foundation. This is foundation sprayed on the skin using an airbrush instead of being apply with conventional tools such as your fingers, a sponge, or a brush. It is a liquid and is released in a fine spray from the end of the spray gun (airbrush), giving the entire face complete coverage. This formula is known for its long wearability. Some formulas are water-resistant and some are waterproof. Because of the complete coverage aspect of it, it can create a mask-like effect.

aerosol spray foundation. This formula comes in an aerosol spray can. It gives you maximum coverage with staying power. Most formulas work on all skin types and are water-resistant. It was created to mimic what professional makeup artists call airbrushing (using a machine that sprays a fine mist of foundation). You simply spray it over your face, and it releases a mist of foundation, giving you complete coverage. After you spray it on, you can use a sponge or a brush to blend it in and help it look more natural. But it tends to look less natural and heavier than many of your other foundation options.

concealer

Concealer can be your best friend or your worst enemy. It comes in a multitude of formulations and textures. Different textures of concealers are used on different problem areas, so it's important to match the texture with the problem area. For example, a concealer used to cover under-eye areas should always be moist and creamy, whereas a concealer designed to cover breakouts or broken capillaries should be much drier in texture so it will adhere better and last longer. If you use the wrong formula, it could draw more attention to what you are trying to conceal.

stick concealers. These full-coverage concealers can vary in dryness and texture; some are creamier and some are much less moist. They conceal everything from dark circles to more prominent blemishes and almost every skin discoloration. When using this formula to minimize under-eye circles, make sure the texture and consistency are creamy enough to blend well and keep the area hydrated so as not to accentuate fine lines. Because your most delicate skin is under your eyes, using a creamier texture will help keep this area looking its most flawless. If you are covering other types of spots on you face, such as blemishes, dark spots, or veins, choose a stick that is a little drier in texture so it will stay put and last longer.

pot concealer. This concealer provides similar full coverage to stick, but it is usually formulated with more moisturizing ingredients and is not quite as thick. It conceals any flaws you might want to hide. This is the concealer most commonly used by professionals because of its great coverage and versatility. There are many formulas out there, some drier and some with more moisture, so find the one that best fits your needs. Although usually creamy, it is also available in drier, oil-free formulas that are used to cover discoloration on the rest of the face (because the drier it is, the better it will adhere and longer it wears).

tube concealer. This has creamier texture than some other formulas. Tube concealer covers dark under-eye circles because it's so moist, and it's one of the easiest to blend. It will probably not have quite the staying power of some other (drier) formulas, so it may not be the best choice for other spots and discoloration. It provides terrific coverage and can be mixed with moisturizer or foundation to create a much sheerer product.

wand concealer. This option offers you one of the lightest and sheerest textures of all concealer formulas. These concealers give you the least coverage, but they blend in most easily and look very natural. They will sometimes settle into fine lines if not completely blended (due to the nature of the texture). If the proper shade is used, you may apply it without a foundation because it will blend so easily into bare skin. A lot of these formulas now contain light-reflecting particles to help disguise imperfections, making up for their lesser coverage with just as much camouflage. Wand concealers provide a quicker, slightly denser coverage than liquid foundation, but less than most other concealer formulas, and they are fabulous for a fast repair (because they're convenient to carry). Some dry to a powder finish that is great for covering facial blemishes because the powder clings, making it longer wearing.

pencil concealer. These concealers effectively cover tiny imperfections such as broken capillaries, blemishes, veins, and any other tiny flaws. You simply draw it on—draw it all along a vein or draw it right on a blemish or any other spots. With an exact color match, flaws can be pinpointed without a lot of blending. Their dry texture helps their long wearability, as well as giving them great staying power. Pencil concealers are also terrific for fixing lip lines. Use it around the outer edge of your lips to erase your natural lip line (so that you can draw on your new one) or prevent lip color from bleeding. No other formula compares to the convenience in carrying this product with you.

oil-free compact. These concealer formulations are best used on the face to hide pimples and spots. They are usually of a longer wearing, drier texture that will not irritate breakouts and will stay right where you put them. Because of their long wearability, they effectively cover age spots and hyperpigmentation (any type of spot on the face). But keep in mind that because of their dry texture, they are the wrong choice for covering under-eye dark circles; they will make the area appear dry and cakey.

highlighting pen. This amazing product contains light-refracting particles, which reflect light to bring forward recessed areas of the face and hide minor flaws. This is not a concealer; it's a highlighter (I stress this because many people are confused about the pen's usage). Everywhere you use it will come forward visually, making it appear even with the rest of the face. In other words, it highlights (brings out) recessed areas, such as the dark shadows created by bags, wrinkles, deep creases, and the inside corners of your eyes. You simply apply it to the shadowed area and it brightens it, making it appear less distinct.

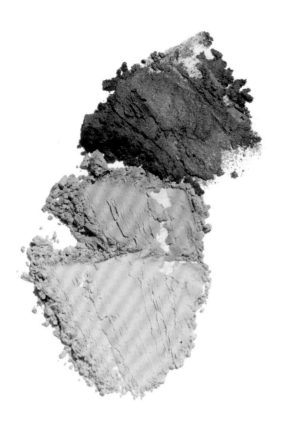

powder

Your makeup will not last the day unless you set it, and that is what powder does for you: it sets everything in place. If you don't powder, when you apply your color products, they will catch on different areas of the skin and look blotchy instead of going on evenly and smoothly. Powder is the finishing step that helps the skin appear smooth and natural. You can even brush it on over a clean, moisturized face for a fresh, no-makeup look.

Powder comes in two basic forms: loose and pressed. Both will set your makeup and absorb excess shine and oil. Loose powder is more oil-absorbing than pressed powder. I always prefer to use loose powder when I am first setting foundation and concealer. It gives a better finish and prevents the need for touch-ups longer. Pressed powder is wonderful because it is easy to carry and use for touch-ups throughout the day. If you have oily skin, powder is a must because it prevents excess shine from the oils in your skin, which can draw attention to textural flaws.

Your powder should be milled as fine as possible. The finer a powder is milled, the higher the quality and the less likely it is to cake on the skin. Finer-milled powders will feel more like velvet, whereas less-milled powders feel grittier.

eyebrows

I find that most people benefit from some brow color. You may not need a lot of filling in, but some will help define and perfect your brow. Each type of brow color will give you more complete coverage or a softer, more natural effect. Choose the formula that helps you fill in slightly or replace what is just not there.

eyebrow pencil. Pencil is the most precise and most common formula used to define the brows. It will give you full coverage and color. It usually has a slightly waxier consistency than other makeup pencils to help it adhere better to the brows and last longer. Formulas that are a little drier and harder give the most natural application. The more strokes you make, the more natural the application will look. Eyebrow pencils come in two forms, mechanical and wood. A mechanical pencil (if it is a good one) will not need to be sharpened. Simply twist it; the product will extend out, and you can apply away. If your pencil is wood, you control the point. Sharpen it before each use. The sharper the point, the better the application.

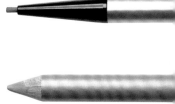

crème. This is the most dramatic-looking brow color. It gives you full coverage when trying to fill in and define your eyebrows. It is a matte crème that is applied with a narrow, stiff-angled eyebrow brush, and it is best to set it with eyebrow powder so it will last and not smudge. I find that it's the least natural-looking option. Even when set with eyebrow powder, it still can smudge, especially on oily skin. If you are a novice or want a subtle look, this is not your best choice.

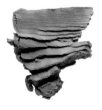

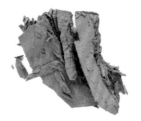

powder. Powder brow color is a matte, no-shimmer powder with a very high pigment content. Powder provides the most natural look when filling in your eyebrows. It is all you need when you are just filling in slightly—maybe the shape of your brow is there, but it's sparse and you need to add a little bulk. In this case, powder is the ideal choice because it will look totally natural, not like you just drew your brows on. It is usually applied with a narrow stiff-angle eyebrow brush (see page 35). It can be used to set brow crèmes, and it helps give pencils even more coverage and lasting power when you are creating a brow from nothing. I often layer powder with pencil for more coverage and more precise application.

pomade. Pomade is a matte, creamy, long-lasting, usually water-resistant brow color. It creates a very dramatic look, much like crème brow color without the smudging and smearing. It's great if you need a lot of filling in because it gives such complete coverage. It controls wild hairs while adding color and giving coverage. Because it is smudge-proof and matte, it does not have to be set with powder, but I do like to follow it with a little powder color to soften the look of it.

brow gel. This is basically a hair gel (or hair spray) for the eyebrows. If your brows seem to look out of place and don't lie perfectly, gel can keep them where you want them. Brow gels are available in tinted or clear formulas. The tinted formulas (also called brow mascara) will not necessarily fill your brows in, but they will make the hairs you do have look fuller and more noticeable, which might be all you want or need, while keeping everything in place. The clear formulas can help set the color (pencil or powder) you already applied, while keeping your eyebrow hairs in place. I am not a big fan of the tinted versions, but I love the clear to keep brows looking great all day.

mascara

How could you live without mascara? You shouldn't. It's the most important element of your eye makeup because of the definition it creates. Full, thick, dark eyelashes help open up your eyes and make you look your absolute best.

Multiple formulas will give you a variety of results. Of course, your application technique will also make a difference in your results (see page 136). Choose the formula that will help you achieve the look you want.

thickening mascara. This mascara coats each individual lash from root to tip with particles that add bulk and help them look thick and full. It is formulated with dark pigments, thicker waxes, and silicone polymers, which are what create the density. This formula is the thickest of all formulas because the goal is to increase lash size. Yes, sometimes size really does matter!

lengthening mascara. This contains plastic polymers that cling to the tips of your eyelashes, making them appear longer. This formula is thinner than a thickening formula, so it will not add the bulk.

defining mascara. Defining mascara coats each individual lash, keeping them separated and defined. If a mascara is labeled as defining, it usually means that it does not contain any extra building particles that add bulk and length to your eyelashes; it simply coats each lash with color for subtle definition. Defining mascara usually appears the most natural.

waterproof mascara. When something is labelled waterproof mascara, the formula has been shown not to smudge or smear when subjected to (submerged or totally dowsed in) water or tears in tests. Most formulas of mascara are available in a waterproof formula. It's a bit harder to remove than other formulas, so make sure you have a good eye-makeup remover for cleansing.

water-resistant mascara. Water-resistant mascara will hinder smearing and smudging, but not as fully as waterproof formulas. It resists rather than entirely preventing the penetration of water, while being easier to remove than waterproof.

curling mascara. This mascara is supposed to help curl your eyelashes as you apply it. The theory is that they contain polymers that contract (shrink) once applied, causing your eyelashes to curl and lift. I have not found these mascaras to do enough curling to get the benefits you need and prevent you from needing to use an eyelash curler.

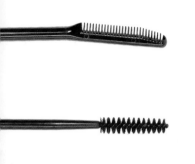

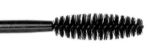

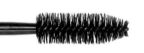

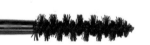

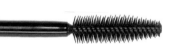

choosing a mascara wand

The bristles and shape of your mascara wand can affect your results just as much as your mascara's formula and your application technique. There are a ton of wand options out there today—everything from a rubber brush to a comb. Let's discuss just a few key things to consider when deciding what you want and need from your brush or applicator. But keep in mind that, with any wand, you still ultimately have control of your finished look because it depends on the application technique you choose. (See page 136.)

- A wand that has long, fat, full, thick, dense bristles will help thicken and lengthen your eyelashes as you apply your mascara because it will coat each lash with product.

- A wand with short, dense bristles (it might even resemble a screw) will help define your eyelashes because it allows you to coat each lash with a nice thin coat of product from the root to the tip.

- A wand with bristles that taper from short at the tip to longer in the middle or base (it might also taper from thin to thick to thin, like a foot-ball), will define, thicken, and lengthen. It enables you to do detailed defining work with the tip (where the tip bristles are shorter), while giving you volume and length from the bristles in the middle (where the bristles are longer and fuller).

- A wand with rubber, widely spaced bristles will define and separate your eyelashes, giving you a thin, even coating on every lash.

- A wand shaped like a comb will define and separate each lash. It will give you a thin coat of product while combing and separating each lash, eliminating clumping and preventing eyelashes from getting stuck together.

tip: *It's always better to apply multiple thin coats of mascara rather than one thick, clumpy coat.*

eyeliner

Eyeliner is an option, not a have-to, when applying your makeup. There are definite benefits to wearing eyeliner, but only if you choose the right formula for your desired effect. Badly applied eyeliner will make you look harsh and make your eyes appear smaller, whereas properly applied eyeliner will open up your eyes, making them look bigger.

pencil eyeliner. Pencil is the most commonly used eyeliner, simply because it is the easiest to control and mistakes are easy to fix. There are many pencil textures available. Some are drier and harder, and some are creamier and glide on effortlessly. In the past, many people felt the need to soften their hard, dry pencils with a lighter or a match. Thankfully, most pencils now contain silicone, which enables them to glide on smoothly and makes them easy to smudge and blend. The best choice is a pencil with just enough silicone to glide on easily, but not so much that it smears or travels. Make sure your pencil is at least water-resistant, so it will stay put and not smudge. Pencils come in both mechanical and wood formulas. A mechanical pencil might not need to be sharpened, depending on the brand; simply twist it so the product extends out and apply. If your pencil is wood, you control the point. Sharpen it before each use to get the best application. The sharper the point, the better the application.

liquid eyeliner. This is a colored liquid that is applied with a fine-tip applicator for precision. You will find multiple applicator options, depending on the brand and formula—everything from a fine-tipped brush (the most common) to a felt-tip pen to a pointed, sponge-tip applicator. Liquid liner is usually long-wearing and looks the most dramatic. Because of this, it might not be the best choice for you if you want to create a soft definition along your top lash line. Liquid liner is a good choice to use after you apply strip false eyelashes because you can successfully conceal the band with it. Liquid eyeliner should only be applied along the top lash line, never along the bottom lash line, where it looks too harsh and unnatural.

tip: *You can turn any eye shadow into a liquid-looking eyeliner. Simply dampen your eyeliner brush and it sweep it across your favorite eye shadow.*

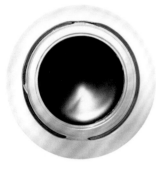

crème or gel eyeliners. These eyeliners are usually packaged in a pot and are applied using a fine-tipped brush. They will give you a similar effect to liquid eyeliner, which means they will appear quite dramatic. Also, because they look much like liquid eyeliner, you should only apply them along the top lash line, never along the bottom lash line, where they will look too harsh and unnatural. One big positive is the fact that they dry much quicker than liquid, which makes them much easier to use without smearing them all over the place. They also tend to be very long-wearing.

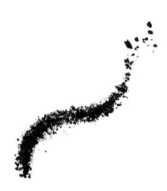

cake eyeliner. Cake eyeliner is a pressed powder–like product that is usually applied with a damp eyeliner brush. It may look like an eye shadow, but it is more heavily pigmented and denser in texture. Most formulas (the more classic versions) work best using a damp brush, but with some formulas, you can use your brush dry. Using a cake formula that works dry will give you a much subtler effect. When applied with a damp brush, it gives you much more dramatic definition. Dampened cake eyeliner will give you a similar effect to liquid eyeliner, but it's much easier to control.

tip: *You can use any powder eye shadow to line with; all you need is the right brush to create the effect you want to achieve. This will give you the most natural and subtle definition along your lash line.*

eye shadow

Eye shadow can do so much to bring attention to your eyes and wake up your face. It can reshape your lids to make them look their most beautiful. When choosing eye shadow, consider both the texture and the finish. Both make an enormous difference in the effect they create and how dramatic they look. Most important, depending on your goals, some choices are better than others. Let's arm you with all the knowledge you need.

texture

powder. These shadows come either loose or pressed. Both formulas vary in finish from matte to shimmer and from iridescent to frosty. The pressed version is the most popular and the easiest to use because it blends so well. Most makeup lines offer the largest color choices in this texture. Loose powder eye shadows (which are usually a purer color pigment) work great and blend as well as their pressed counterparts, but you must be a little more careful of shadow fall-off. (This is no big deal: after dipping your applicator in shadow, just make sure to tap the excess off before you apply). Powder shadows can be applied with a brush, sponge-tip applicator, or your fingers, but a brush gives you the best blend and results.

crème. These shadows are available in every finish; the most popular are shimmers, frosts, and mattes. They are great if you have dry eyelids. Be careful, though, because many crème shadows can crease. However, there are some crème eye shadows that dry to a powder finish. Many, if not most, are at least water-resistant; some are waterproof and long-wearing. For more intense color, layer a crème eye shadow on first and follow it with a powder eye shadow. This will make them harder to blend, so make sure you place the color where you want it when you first apply it.

pencil. These are eye shadows put into a convenient pencil form. They are useful for around the eye, close to the lash line, because they are sharpened to a point and can be applied with precision. They also work great anywhere on the eyelid. Their precision makes it easy to get the product right where you want and need it (whether it be the lash line, crease, or brow bone). After application, simply smudge the line with your finger, a sponge-tip applicator, or a brush to blend and create the effect you want.

liquid. Liquid shadows usually come in a shiny, metallic finish, and they are the hardest to use. Because liquid shadow doesn't blend easily, you must be precise (make sure you get it right where you want it from the start), so it's best when applied with a brush. Liquid is usually used either as an eyeliner or applied close to the lash line for color intensity.

finish

matte. Matte finish has absolutely no shine or shimmer to it. Matte-textured eye shadows are the best for creating a natural, no-makeup look. They usually contain a higher level of color pigment, and they work well for reshaping and defining the eye. A matte finish is the best for mid-tone shades, which need to look very natural. A matte shadow will draw absolutely no attention to any fine lines or crepe-like texture on your eyelids.

shimmer. Shimmer shadows have a subtle sheen and give a hint of sparkle. They offer great, sheer coverage; when you sweep on the color, you can still see the skin underneath. They usually contain multiple shades of mica (the shiny particle) that are sheer and transparent, softening their appearance on the skin. Because the mica is see-through, it is less likely to collect in fine lines. Light shimmer shadows work great for highlighting and bringing out recessed areas of the eyelid. Dark shimmer shadows are ideal for adding drama without being as harsh and intense as matte shades because the shimmer particles reflect light and soften the final effect.

satin. Satin shadows fall in between matte and shimmer. They are shinier than a matte, but have no sparkle or shimmer to them, so they give the eyelid a sheen without appearing sparkly or glittery. They are great for dry lids to create a natural look without turning as ashy as a matte shadow might. A satin finish is easy to wear and works well on all skin types.

frosted. Frosted shadows have the absolute most shine or sheen to them. They can actually look reflective. A frosted eye shadow gives you a much opaquer coverage than a shimmer shadow, completely covering the skin underneath it. The mica (the shiny particle) in a frost is usually one shade, most often a silvery white, and each little fleck of mica is opaque as well. Because of this, they create the most drama and change in color when used, but the little flecks of mica can collect in fine lines and draw more attention to them. They usually come in fun, light pastel shades as well as great metallic shades.

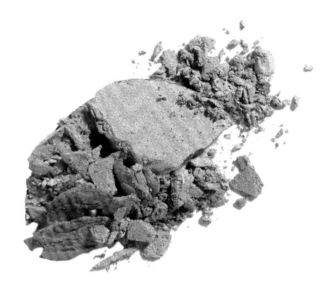

blush

Blush can be one of your best friends or, again, one of your worst enemies if chosen wrong. It can bring a gorgeous glow to your cheeks and give you an amazing sexy flush. But because some people find it hard to use correctly, they just steer clear of it.

The formula, texture, and finish can make the biggest difference in whether your blush is your friend or your enemy. Most textures of blush come in multiple finishes, from matte and shimmer. Some formulas are easier than others to apply and use, while some have a much greater staying power. Different formulas also can give you differing degrees of coverage; some are sheer and some contain heavier pigments, giving you more coverage and intensity of color.

powder. Powder blush is color pigment set in a powder base. It's the most popular type of blush because it's the easiest to control and use, and therefore, it's usually available in the widest range of shades. Applied with a soft blush brush, it gives a dusting of color that works well with the majority skin types. Powder blush is the best choice for oily skin, but if you have really dry skin, this formula might not be your best friend. It's wonderful for combination and normal skin. It is usually packaged in a pressed form (the most convenient and easy to carry), but can also be found in a loose version. Some formulas are matte, and some contain shimmer. The matte version tends to look the most natural and will not accentuate textural flaws in your skin.

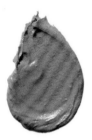

crème. This blush is color pigment set in a crème base. It has a fresh dewy finish that gives the face a luminous, natural glow. It is great for normal to dry skin, but an especially good choice for dry skin because it slides easily over the surface and blends into the skin. It works best when applied after your foundation and before your powder so it can blend in more easily. Unfortunately, if you have oily skin, crème blush is not your best choice because it will not wear well. And it does not work well on skin with large pores because it tends to accentuate them. It's great for those who do not need or want to wear foundation. Just apply it with your fingers, a sponge, or the appropriate brush and work it into your skin. You can also layer it under powder blush for more intense color and longer wear.

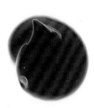

gel. Gel blush contains color pigments wrapped within silicone particles. It works best on people with normal to dry skin because it won't last on oily skin. It smooths nicely onto bare skin to create a pretty, sheer, translucent glow. That's not to say you can't use it with foundation; you can. Just make sure you apply it before you powder. It is long-lasting, looks natural, and is easy to use. You can use your fingers or a sponge to apply it and then smooth it into the skin.

liquid. This blush or tint is a liquid that stains the skin temporarily. It works on all skin types. It is applied like the gel blush, but it's a little more difficult to work with—it must be blended quickly due to its staining quality. (Practice will make perfect!) It's waterproof, so you can expect it to last all day. Just like with gel blush, you can use either a sponge or your fingers to apply it and blend it into your skin.

bronzer

Bronzer is the secret to having an eternal glow. Everyone can benefit from it. I do not think I have ever applied makeup to anyone's face and not used bronzer. Bronzers also come in multiple textures and finishes, and choosing the right formula is the key to achieving the desired effect.

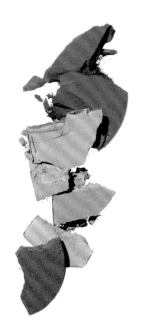

powder. Like powder blush, powder bronzer is easy to control and blend. It comes pressed into a compact, loose in a tub, or even pressed into small balls or beads in a jar. This formula works on most skin types (normal, combination, and oily), but it might not be your best choice if you have very dry skin. Powder bronzers vary in finishes from matte to a heavy dose of shimmer. In most cases, I choose a matte finish (except for really dark skin tones; a little shimmer can give you a glow) because I think it looks the most natural. Also, because bronzer covers such a large area of your face, too much shimmer could draw attention to textural flaws. Swept across strategic areas of the face with a brush, it can bring the skin to life.

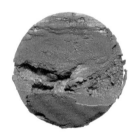

crème. Like bronzing powder, crème bronzer is used to give your face a sun-kissed glow. You can find it in a stick or even in compacts. This formula works best on normal to dry skin, especially dry. It comes in a multitude of finishes, from matte to shimmer. Make sure you apply it after your foundation and before you powder so it blends beautifully. It's also a good choice when you don't want to wear foundation but want that little extra glow because it will blend beautifully onto bare skin. It can be applied with your fingers, a sponge, or a foundation brush.

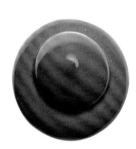

gel. Gel bronzer, like powder and crème, will help give you that sun-kissed glow. This formula works best on normal to dry skin. The main difference is that it will give you a much sheerer wash of color. This is basically a sheer gel containing color pigments, which makes it very easy to blend into the skin. If you are trying to cover a large area of skin (legs, arms, or body), this formula will be the easiest to apply and blend. Most often, this formula comes packaged in a tube. It comes in multiple finishes. Always apply it before any powder products so it will blend well.

lip color

Lip color is so personal. One formula does not work for everyone. Some people want a lot of coverage and moisture from their lipstick or gloss, while others just want a sheer wash of color that looks and feels like it isn't even there. You will find a variety of textures of lipstick and lip glosses out there, with a variety of finishes. Play, test, and try until you find what you like. But keep in mind that moisture is always good for your lips; it keeps them full and supple-looking.

matte lipstick. Matte lipstick delivers sophisticated and intense full coverage with absolutely no shine. Because of its formulation, it stays on longer than other lipsticks, but it can be drying and may give your lips the feeling and appearance of being dehydrated. With up-to-date technology, there are now some matte formulas that are not quite so dry and dehydrating, but they will not last as long as drier versions. Matte lipsticks are great in dark, intense shades because they stay put and won't smear very easily. You can always make a matte lipstick appear more luscious by applying a lip gloss on top.

crème lipstick. This contains more emollients than matte lipstick and provides a full coverage of moist (though not shiny) color. Most cosmetic lines offer the largest selection in this formula because it is the most versatile and popular. It wears quite well without being as dehydrating as matte lipstick. Keep in mind that there will still be different degrees of moisture in crème lipsticks, depending on the formulation and the brand. Crème formulas can have a natural, frosted, or shimmer finish, and the finish you choose can dramatically affect how your lips appear.

sheer or glaze lipsticks. These give you a glossy, sheer wash of see-through color that allows your natural lips to show through because they are not formulated to cover opaquely. This formula contains color pigments wrapped in a transparent hydrating gel, adding color while making your lips feel moist and full. The coverage will last longer than a gloss, but not as long as a crème lipstick. It's terrific for a quick fix because due to its sheerness, it doesn't have to be applied with precision.

long-wearing lipstick. Long-wearing lipstick is a heavily pigmented, usually very matte, formula with a dry texture so it stays put and is long lasting. It will almost stain the lips with very full coverage and very drying and dehydrating. I personally hate these formulas because they tend to make your lips look smaller and shriveled. Luscious full lips are always more beautiful, and this formula will not make that happen. Some formulas will come with a gloss to wear on top to combat the negative effects. But this cuts down on their wearability because anytime you add moisture it shortens the life of a lipstick.

frost. This finish provides a shiny, metallic appearance to a lipstick. The metallic appearance is created from small flecks of a shine-producing material, which are solid and reflective, mixed into the lipstick formula. A high concentration of these particles gives more opaque coverage and can make the lips appear a bit dry. They're not the best choice giving your lips a luscious pout! They are good when used for layering on top of a satin-finished lipstick to lighten up the depth of a shade.

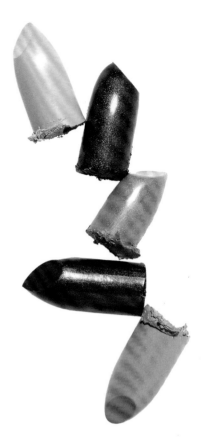

shimmer. This finish provides a beautiful, lustrous, glowing appearance to a lipstick. This finish is created by mixing tiny particles that produce shine into the formula. The difference between frost and shimmer is that the particles used in a shimmer finish are not opaque—they are sheer and see-through, so they just create a glow without being extremely reflective. There are also multiple colors of these reflective particles instead of a single color, like in a frosted formula. They have a nice, easy-to-wear, medium amount of coverage and can make lips look fuller.

gloss. This lip product adds extreme shine and moisture to your lips. I love lip gloss, mainly because it immediately adds fullness and makes your lips look kissable. It delivers a sheer to medium layer of color coverage. The only problem is that it does not have a very long wear life, so it is going to need frequent reapplication. Although it doesn't last terribly long, gloss gives a fresh-and-alive look to all age groups. Used correctly, it can make the lips look fuller and sexier. You'll find it packaged in a wand, tube, or pot. Some formulas do give more coverage than others and some formulas now also offer longer-wear, (still a gloss; consider the source), so test drive a few to find a formula or brand that will give you what you need. Some key words that might give you a clue to the wear time: luster, lacquer, gel, plastic, rich, or glass could mean longer wear life, while crystal, wet, transparent, glaze, or juicy could mean a high shine factor but probably shorter wear time. Play away!

lip liner. Lip liner is a pencil that helps define and reshape your lips. It helps correct your lips' shape, as well as prevent lip color from bleeding into fine lines. It can also be used over the entire lip, and then topped with a lipstick or lip gloss. Either way, a layer of lip liner greatly improves the staying power of any lip color. Lip liner comes in two forms: mechanical and wood. A mechanical pencil might not need to be sharpened; simply twist, the product will extend out, and you can apply away. If your pencil is wood, you control the point; just sharpen it before each use because the sharper the point, the better the application.

essential tools

As with anything that you do in life, using the right tools to apply makeup will make your job much easier. Let's go through a variety of makeup tools: what they do, what makes some better than others, what to look for when buying them, and how to use them. For all the tools in this chapter, visit www.robertjonesbeauty.com to get what you need.

brushes

There are so many shapes, sizes, and types of brushes out there that it can become confusing when choosing. Unfortunately, price does make a difference: the better brushes are more expensive. Brushes in makeup artists' lines tend to be designed better and give you better shape options. Also, different brush head shapes make a difference in the effect they create.

Here are some key points to consider when choosing your brushes:

- **The bristle.** There are several types of bristles, from natural to synthetic, and each can make a difference in your application. For powder, you will always get better application from a natural bristle because the cuticles on the hair pick up and lay down the particles of the powder better than a synthetic bristle. With a crème product, most times you will use a synthetic bristle so it doesn't absorb the moisture from the product. Let's discuss all the options:

  - **squirrel.** The highest quality, most expensive option, squirrel is a natural bristle, so it gives you an even, smooth application. It's used for powder products, not crème. It is the softest of all the bristle choices. Many companies, including mine, have stopped using squirrel because no factory can guarantee that the animal is not killed in harvesting its hair for the brushes. For all other hair types, the animals are just given a haircut.

  - **pony.** A pony bristle is one step below squirrel in quality. It is often used for powder and blush brushes because of its length, but can also be used to create other brushes. A natural bristle, it's used for the application of powder products dry. Even though the name may not suggest it, this bristle feels quite soft.

- **sable.** Sable is a high-quality bristle, one step down from pony. It is commonly used in the creation of eye shadow brushes; it's rarely used for larger brushes because of its length. This is also a natural bristle, so it will give an even, blended application. It's most often used for the application of powder products dry, but it can be used wet or damp for application of crèmes. Using it while damp is not the best choice when applying foundation. Because it's a natural bristle, it will absorb all the liquid from your foundation.

- **black silk.** This is the next level down, but there are many levels of quality black silk products, even some as high quality as squirrel. It is actually a treated version of goat hair that makes it feel softer and smoother in its application. A natural bristle, it's best when used dry with powder products.

- **goat.** Goat is the least expensive natural bristle used in making brushes. Thanks to its cost and wide availability, it's the most commonly used of all the natural bristles. It's often used for blush and bronzer brushes because of its length and cost-effectiveness. Sable hairs are too short to be used for longer-bristled brushes, so often goat hairs are used in their place; for example, in blush, powder, and bronzer brushes. Like the other natural-bristle brushes, it's used for applying powder products dry. Some treated goat bristles, however, can be used for creme, liquid, and foundation application. Because of the size of their cuticles, they will not absorb all the liquid, making them a great tool.

- **synthetic.** A synthetic bristle is specifically designed for applying liquid and crème products. It will not absorb the moisture or liquid out of a product. It can be used to apply powder products as well, but it will not do as good a job as a natural bristle due to its lack of cuticles to grab and distribute the powder. This is the best bristle choice for foundation, concealer, and many eyeliner brushes because of its compatibility with crèmes and liquids and its ability to be used damp. It is also easy to clean, yet another reason it works well for foundation and concealer brushes.

- **The handle.** Make sure you choose a handle shape that feels comfortable in your hand. It's key to how easy a brush is for you to use. I find that shorter handles work better. If they are too long, they never pack easily and can cause the brush to feel off balance in your hand. The extra length gets in the way.

- **The head shape.** The contour and shape of the head of a brush makes all the difference in how it applies a product. The length, the tapering of the hairs, density, quality, and stiffness all affect application. Shorter, denser hairs give you more precise application, although you still want tapered ends to prevent lines. Longer, more flexible eye shadow brush bristles will give you a softer application of color. Eye shadow blending brushes are longer, softer, and more flexible to allow you to blend color without completely removing it. Blush and bronzer brushes need to be very dense and full, while again staying flexible, for more color deposit and a softer blended application. An eyebrow brush needs bristles that are stiffer and compact for a more precise placement of color. Concealer brushes need to come to a bit of a point for exact application. The ends of eyeliner brushes are usually flatter and blunter to create an exact line.

get the shape you need

I've used practically every type of brush out there. If it's been created, I've tried it. I love brushes. I truly believe that with the right tool, you can create anything, and having the right tool can mean the difference in whether what you are trying to do even ends up looking anything like you intended. I have spent years perfecting the shape of each one of these brushes to make application more foolproof. Because again, with the right tool, a novice can look like a pro. This collection of brushes will give you everything you need for every makeup application. I will also call out the numbers throughout the book during application to help you understand usage and application techniques. They are always available on www.robertjonesbeauty.com.

eyebrow/eyelash brushes

#1. This is the perfect brush for applying color and shaping your eyebrows. Its short, stiff bristles and narrow angle will give you an exact application. The firmness of this brush is vital to its ability to give precise placement of color. The edges of the angle are also tapered for softness of color and to help blend. It's traditionally used for application of eyebrow powder and crème brow color, but it's also your best friend for blending eyebrow pencil once applied.

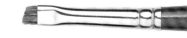

brow brush. I know it may look like a toothbrush, but it's not. It's for grooming and shaping your eyebrows and for trimming brows because of it can brush the entire brow. It's also great for blending everything after all color applications, softening it and making it look more natural.

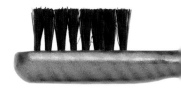

eyelash comb #3. An eyelash comb is a must for your eyelashes. After applying mascara, combing your eyelashes will help separate every lash while removing any clumps. The fine metal teeth allow exact precision (its plastic counterpart can't get the separation that the metal teeth can).

eye shadow brushes

#11. This tapered, natural-bristle brush expertly applies your favorite midtone shade in the crease with precision, from the outer corner of your eye to the inside corner. The shape helps apply your color right where you want it while helping blend it. It can also be used as a blending brush, due to the length of its bristles and their softness.

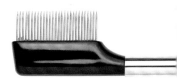

#20. Don't be fooled by this brush's large size. Its precisely tapered, natural bristles are amazing for creating exact creases. It allows you to get the right placement while its soft beveled bristles create the perfect crease. It's the go-to brush for eye shapes, such as deep-set eyes, for which you really need complete control of your midtone.

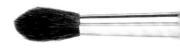

#14. This sable brush is for applying your highlight shade at the inside corner of your eye and the lower lash line (which you will discover opens the eyes for a wide-eyed look). You can also use it for smudging liner and detailed color application.

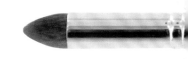

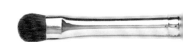

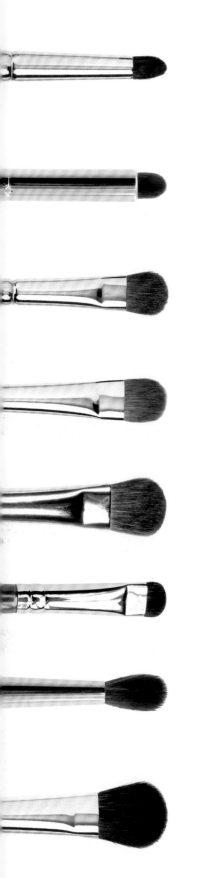

#13. This is a miracle brush you shouldn't be without. Its precision-shaped, natural bristles are perfect for applying your favorite shade of eye shadow along the lower lash line while giving you a smudged and blended effect with no harsh lines. You can also use it for creating a very defined line of color in the crease of the eye (creating a cut crease).

#19. This is the ultimate smudging brush. Made of natural bristles, its shape is beveled, with a slightly blunt end, allowing you to smudge your color as you apply it, never creating any harsh lines. Its unique shape is also perfect for using after you've applied color with another brush to smudge it out.

#30. This precision brush, made of pony hair with the edges tapered for blending, is for applying your most intense shade of eye shadow along the lash line and into the outer corner of the crease of the eye. Its shape is ideal for creating a wide variety of looks and effects.

#22. This sable eye shadow brush is for precisely applying a highlight shade to your brow bone and eyelid. It's also a go-to brush for applying color anywhere whenever you want a brush with a slightly stiffer feel. Because of its bristle shape and texture, it works perfectly for crème shadows.

#27. This natural-bristle brush is the perfect size and shape for applying color over a large area of your lid. Its long, soft bristles give you ultimate flexibility and makes it the must-have tool for creating a smoky eye.

#38. This brush's natural bristles are a shorter length and beveled to give you great control, whether you use it to apply a shadow as a smudged liner or to smudge out your pencil. It's perfect for controlled blending.

#16. This detailed blending brush is made from the softest natural bristles. The long length of the bristles, with their slightly blunt end, blend your shadows while keeping everything very detailed. The only way to get a perfect blend with your eye shadows is to have a clean brush that you use just for blending, and this is that brush. It's a must-have for detail freaks.

#28. This super soft, natural-bristle brush is perfect for all-over blending. It's a must when you're wearing more than one eye color. Keep this brush free of color so you can use it to blend multiple shades.

tip: *When applying a powder product, use a brush with natural bristles. For crème products, use a brush with synthetic bristles. When applying a crème-to-powder product, you can use either.*

eyeliner brushes

#41. This is my secret weapon for eyes that grab attention; it's a tiny brush with big results. Use this synthetic-bristle brush to push color into your lash line, which makes your eye color really pop and your eyelashes look thick. It's also perfect for very detailed lining.

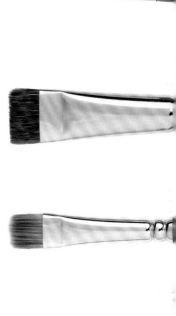

#18. Use this wide, flat, natural-bristle brush to precisely apply a line of bold or soft eye color along the lash line and blend it up onto the lid. It makes your application easy because of its shape; simply lay the brush flat on the lid along your lash line and brush up. It's great for helping you create a smoky eye.

#40. This is a flat, synthetic-bristle brush used to line and define eyes with eye shadow or to apply powder over your pencil liner to create a subtler effect. It is also great for blending your pencil without adding color; simply brush across the pencil you applied to smooth the line. It's perfect for wet or dry use.

#42. This is the perfect liquid/gel eye liner brush because of its shape.

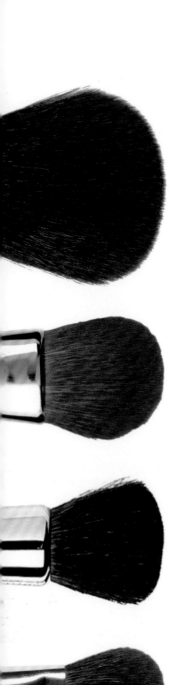

complexion/face-perfecting brushes

#70. This big and fluffy black silk brush is for brushing on loose powder smoothly, giving you sheer, even application. The black silk bristles increase the softness and quality of application. The slightly tapered head shape assists with your application.

#73. This natural-bristle brush is versatile and irreplaceable! So many uses, so little time. Because of its size and beveled shape, it is perfect for loose and pressed powder application, unbelievable for removing excess loose powder after powder puff application, and priceless for very detailed blush and face contour application.

#74. Nothing works better when applying powder foundation than a natural-bristle brush with tapered edges. They prevent streaking and give you even coverage, with the softest application. Don't forget that with a brush like this, size does matter, so you can reach all the detailed areas of the face.

#76. This natural-bristle brush is the ultimate for detail powdering. Because of its shape and size, nothing beats it for powdering in small areas, such as under your eyes and eyelids. There is no better brush for applying powder highlights and face shimmers with precision.

#60. This is the ultimate blush and bronzer brush. It's made with the softest natural bristles, which are the absolute best for applying blush or bronzer. Its full, dense, long bristles, round shape, and expert tapering blend your blush or bronzer for the most professional application.

#64. This apple-popping blush brush is made of the softest, highest quality natural bristles. The round, dense, full, tapered shape applies color to the apples of the cheek without creating any hard or definite edges. It's the perfect shape for applying crème blush, if you don't like using your fingers.

#50. This synthetic-bristle brush is used to apply concealer with exact precision. Its pointed, tapered shape allows you to cover spots or flawed areas of the face without over-blending or overworking your concealer. Without this brush, you can't cover the tiny flaws that you want to disappear. A concealer brush is an absolute must-have.

#53. This updated pointed shape is amazing for concealing. This synthetic-bristle brush is perfection for concealing larger areas or in curved areas of your face, like under your eyes and around your nose. Talk about fast, perfect application!

#54. Use this tapered, pointed, synthetic-bristle brush to apply crème or liquid foundation. It gives a smooth, even application, producing a flaw-less finish to your skin. It's the first foundation brush that works for stippling. And it's the best tool for end-of-the-day touch-ups, when you don't want to start over but need a fix.

#58. This custom-made natural-bristle flat brush head allows you to buff foundation onto your skin. It distributes pigments evenly, creating a totally flawless, air-brushed finish. It also works well for women with acne, large pores, scarring, or rosacea because it doesn't force the foundation into the pores, but instead brushes over them. It bristles are perfect for crème-to-powder foundation.

#59. This brush has luxuriously soft, densely packed natural bristles arranged in an oval shape. Nicknamed "the stippling brush," it's the go-to brush for applying and stippling out your concealer. It's the perfect brush for shading or blending creamy or powdery products.

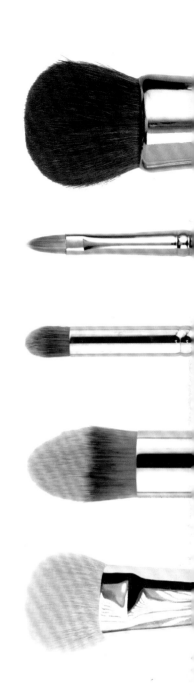

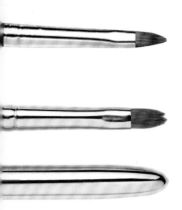

lip brushes

#80. Use this lip brush with a fine tapered point for applying lipstick and lip gloss with precision. If you apply lipstick with a brush, it will last longer, and if you apply lip gloss with a brush, it will look shinier.

#81. This soft sable lip brush with a fine tapered point is perfect for applying lipstick and lip gloss with precision. The benefit of a pull-apart top is that it's perfect for travel or your purse, convenient for touch-ups anytime.

good brush hygiene

You must clean your brushes regularly, or you won't get the application and clarity of color that you want and need. The cleaner the tool, the better the application. You have a couple of cleaning options:

- **brush cleanser.** This option is certainly the simplest; professional brush cleansers work beautifully. Most of them are fast-drying, which makes them even more convenient. You simply dip your brush in the cleanser and wipe it off on a towel, cleaned to perfection.

- **shampoo.** Your other option is to shampoo your brushes. Because brushes are made from hair (natural or synthetic), shampoo works great; it will just take longer for them to dry. A gentle baby shampoo works best and will not be too harsh. Just dampen your brush, and then, with a bit of shampoo in the palm of your hand, work the brush in a circular motion into the shampoo and rinse. I find it best to lightly condition and rinse the brushes after washing. A light leave-in hair conditioner works best because it is very lightweight, but be sure to rinse it out; don't leave it in. Just remember not to get the handles wet; wood and water do not mix. Finally, squeeze out all the excess moisture (making sure to reshape the brushes, so that when they dry the shape will be correct) and lay them flat on a towel to dry.

eyelash curler

No matter which option you choose, the goal is the same: to curl your eyelashes, opening up your eyes, making them look bigger and more awake (see page 134).

classic crimp curler. The most widely used, this version is used only before applying mascara, never after. Make sure that the rubber pad or pads have curved edges to create a better curl, not a crimp. Replace your curler at least once a year and the rubber piece at least once every six months.

precision-detailed curler. This curler works like a crimp curler, but its width makes it easier to get at the root of your eyelashes. I use it to curl the far inside and outside corner eyelashes that most crimp curlers miss. It is easier to use on short eyelashes. It's the only lash curler that works for certain eye shapes, such as deep-set eyes, which a classic crimp curler cannot get into the socket and to the base of the eyelashes.

heated curler. This miracle product is a must-have! It works after you apply your mascara. If you try to use a crimp or precision-detailed curler after applying mascara, it could rip eyelashes out and cause clumping. The heated curler uses the mascara as a curling catalyst, which helps the curl last all day. This curler will curl even the most stubborn eyelashes that no other curler will.

tweezers

Good-quality tweezers are the only way to get your eyebrows perfectly shaped. Get a pair with slanted tips, which will allow you to be as detailed as needed and get every little hair without the danger of injury. Good-quality tweezers can be sharpened when they become dull and will no longer reach the smallest hairs. (The packaging will usually give you an address to which you can send them to be sharpened.)

sponges

When choosing a sponge, consider the texture and quality. The better the quality, the better-looking the application. Price can definitely matter. Different shapes make it easier to get makeup where you want it. The material a sponge is made from will also affect the application.

Today, you have many choices: your traditional triangular wedge, oval, and round sponges. One of my latest favorite tools is a new egg-shaped sponge called the beautyblender. What makes it so amazing is the texture and shape, allowing you to create an airbrushed finish to your foundation. It's also latex free.

powder puff

The best puffs are usually fluffy with a soft velour texture. The beauty of a puff is that it allows you to really push the powder into the skin, creating a smooth, evenly applied, flawless finish. It's a good idea to invest a little more and get a good-quality powder puff so you can launder it to keep it clean. Use it for applying pressed or loose powder.

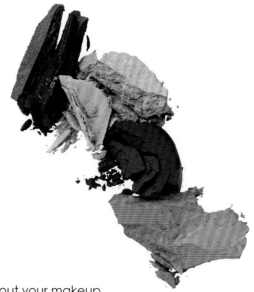

makeup overhaul

If you're a makeup junkie, or if you haven't cleaned out your makeup drawer in years, it's time for an overhaul. I'm willing to bet you have at least some makeup you shouldn't or just don't wear. Time for a fresh start.

On your first pass through your collection, throw out anything you haven't worn in the last year to year and a half. If you haven't used it within that time frame, you're not going to. Plus, colors change in makeup just like they do in fashion, so even if you were to go back to it, it could be out of style.

For your second pass, let's talk real expiration dates. Believe it or not, makeup really does expire—just check out the chart opposite. Use it to decide which products in your makeup drawer and bag to keep and which to toss based on their age. And of course, if a product changes color or starts to smell, it has gone bad. Throw it away.

As you'll see on the chart, some products last much longer than others. Things you put around your eyes that can breed bacteria—such as mascara—need to be changed out much more often. Creamy things that you double dip in should also be changed regularly because they can breed bacteria too. Natural or organic products, because they don't contain any preservatives, go bad relatively quickly. Powders last much longer.

Makeup manufacturers are not by law required to put expiration dates on their products, but most do feature a symbol that tells you how long it's good after being opened. It is a picture of an open jar with a number followed by the letter *m*, for the number of months you have after you open it.

How you store your makeup also makes a difference. Keep it dry and out of the sun and heat. The more temperature controlled you keep it, the longer it will last. If it goes from cold to hot and hot to cold too many times, it can go bad much quicker.

how long does your makeup last?

These timelines are based on makeup industry and health industry recommendations.

product	before opening	after opening
primer	3 years	2 years
foundation: jar, stick, pump, or tube	3 years	1 year
foundation: pot or compact	3 years	6 months
foundation: powder	5 years	2–3 years
concealer: stick, tube, compact, or pot	3 years	1 year
concealer: sponge tip	3 years	6 months
powder	5 years	2–3 years
blush: powder	3 years	2 years
blush: crème	3 years	1 year
bronzer: powder	3 years	2 years
bronzer: crème	3 years	1 year
mascara	3 years	3 months
liquid eyeliner	3 years	3 months
gel eyeliner	3 years	6 months
eye primer	3 years	6 months
eyeliner pencil	6 years	2 years
eye shadow: powder	3 years	2 years
eye shadow: crème	3 years	1 year
brow pencil	6 years	2 years
brow powder	3 years	2 years
brow pomade	3 years	1 year
brow gel	3 years	1 year
lip liner	6 years	2 years
lipstick	3 years	2 years
lip gloss	3 years	2 years
lip balm	3 years	2 years
organic products	6 months	6 months

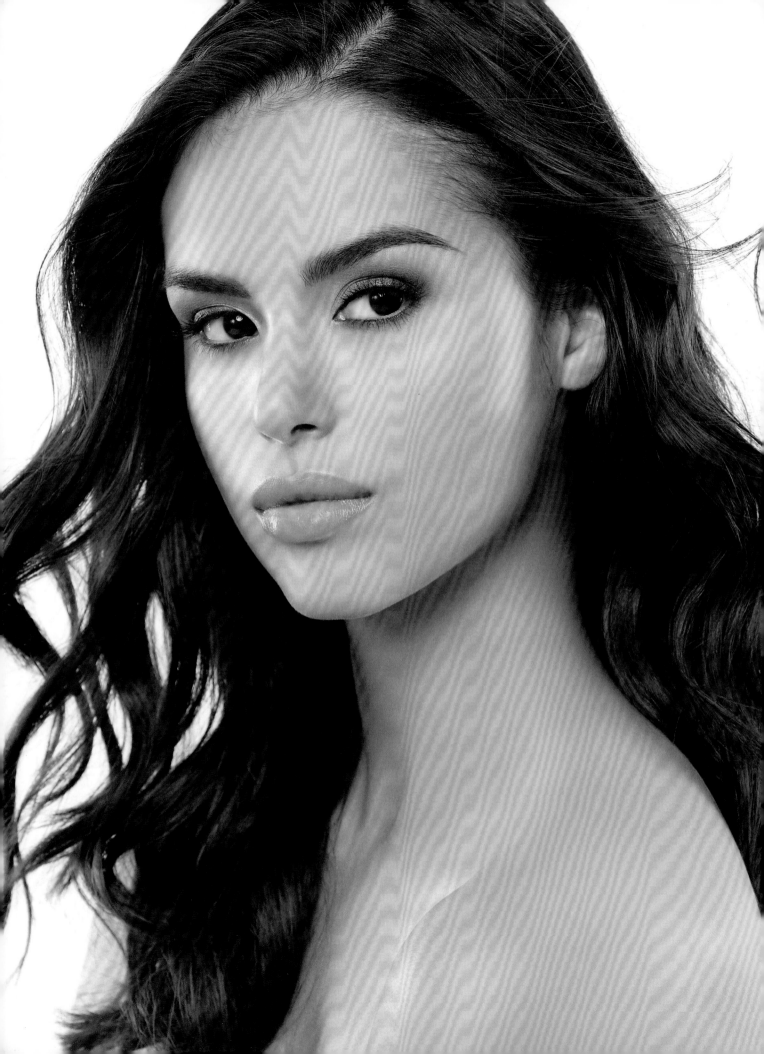

chapter 2

color theory

When it comes to makeup, one of the hardest—and most essential—concepts to understand is color. Yet I find that most people zone out when makeup artists start talking about the color wheel and how it applies to the face.

There are tons of videos and literature on color theory and beauty, but often they don't exactly speak to makeup. I have an artist's background, so my understanding of the color wheel and how it works comes from many, many years of studying art. Color theory in the art world is fascinating, but it's not easy to apply it directly to makeup.

So let's discuss the basics of the color wheel first. Then we'll make it more makeup friendly! I'll show you how to apply those color theory principles. We'll let go of the classic color wheel itself and use a model more specific to our needs. You can use it to choose the colors that work best for you.

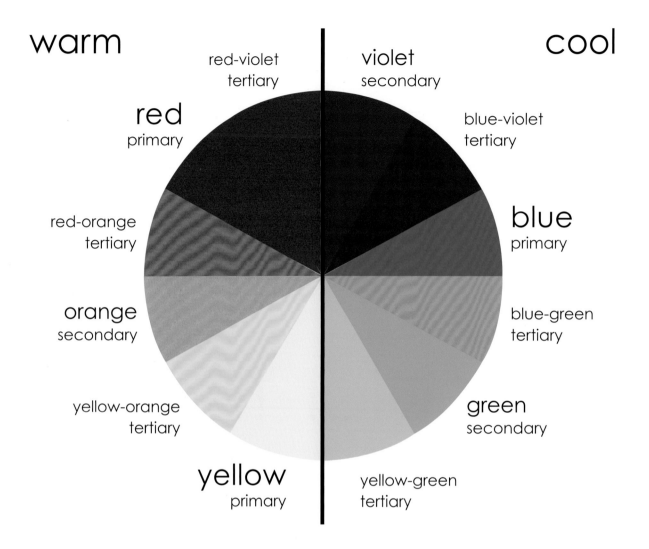

warm

cool

red-violet
tertiary

violet
secondary

red
primary

blue-violet
tertiary

red-orange
tertiary

blue
primary

orange
secondary

blue-green
tertiary

yellow-orange
tertiary

green
secondary

yellow
primary

yellow-green
tertiary

color basics

When you look at a color wheel, you're looking at three different things: primary colors, secondary colors, and tertiary colors. Primary colors are standalone colors—blue, yellow, and red. They cannot be made by mixing other colors.

Secondary colors are mixtures of two primaries. If you mix blue and red together, they make violet. Red and yellow make orange. Yellow and blue make green. Violet, orange, and green are secondary colors.

Tertiary colors are mixtures of a primary and a secondary. Yellow-orange, for example, is a mixture of yellow, a primary, with orange, a secondary. Red-orange and blue-violet are tertiary colors too.

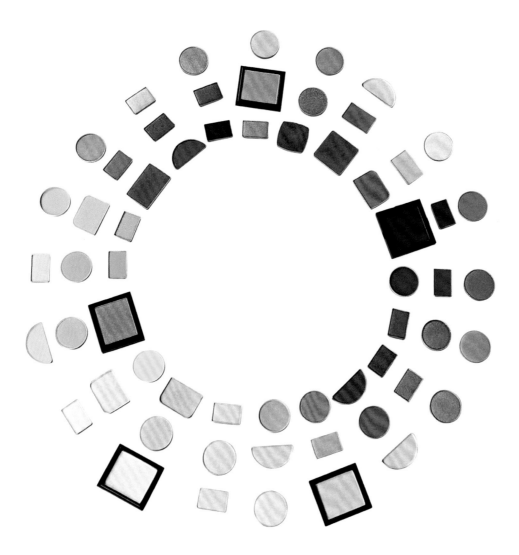

Let's make this easier to see and understand. This color wheel made of eye shadow is more relatable to makeup and easier to understand when talking about beauty. So now when I'm referring to a color, it will be easier to see based on realistic shades that work on the skin.

There's one more characteristic we need to discuss: a color is either cool or warm. A cool shade is blue based, and a warm shade is yellow based. You can have cool and warm versions of almost every shade.

Even colors everyone thinks of as cool can have warm shades: There are cool blues and warm blues, for example. On the color wheel, the middle and right rows ot blue are cool, but in the row to the left, the addition of a little yellow creates warm blues. Likewise, the gray next to the blues is cool, but the gray on the other side of the chart is warm. It's simply a standard gray with some yellow added to warm it up.

eye shadow

The first color choice you'll need to make is for your eye shadow. There are three basic things to think about when choosing eye shadow. The first and most important is your eye color.

You may be used to emphasizing your eye color with clothing, which works differently. If you have blue eyes and you're wearing a blue blouse, that blouse sits at a distance from your eyes, drawing the blue in them out and making them look bluer. But if you put that blue up next to them, it competes with them, making them look less blue. When dealing with eye shadow, you want what we call a complementary opposite: the shade across the color wheel. This was discovered by Leonardo da Vinci: Whenever you pair two opposing colors, they intensify each other.

For instance, let's say you have any shade of blue eyes. If I were to put blue eye shadow on your eyelids, you wouldn't know what to look at first. It would detract from your blue eyes. But if I were to put a bronzy warm color—a shade opposite blue on the color wheel—on your eyelids, it would make your eyes look bluer. You'd look at your eyes first.

So, look for a complementary opposite to bring out your eye color. Anything that's warm will bring out blue, even a burgundy. You can test this: lay a blue in between purple and burgundy. You'll see how the burgundy brings the blue out more than the purple because it has red added to it, making it a warmer shade.

If you have any shade of green eyes, a green eye shadow would, similarly, not accentuate your green. You want a complementary opposite instead. Purple, burgundy, or copper would make your green eyes look greener. Look for colors opposite green on the color wheel on page 46 for shades that enhance green.

If you have brown eyes, you can simply play with color to your heart's content. You can use any shade you want. Keep in mind, though, that some brown eyes might have a little more gold to them. If they do, a warm, coppery shade will bring that gold out. Look across the color wheel for a complementary opposite: Purples will bring that gold out. Greens will not.

What if you have multiple flecks in your eyes? Let's say you have blue eyes with golden flecks. You're going to see mainly blue, and that's what we want to bring out, so look opposite blue on the color wheel. You'll find warm coppery shades and burgundies, colors that will bring out your blue while still enhancing the gold because these shades are complementary opposites of the gold as well. If you have green eyes with golden flecks, look across the color wheel to burgundies, warm browns, and purples. These shades will really bring out that green and that gold.

If you have hazel eyes, you've probably realized that they aren't just one color. They're a mixture of either green and brown or green and blue. If they are green and blue, you get to decide which color you want to bring out more. If you want to bring out the blue, go across from blue to the coppery shades. If you want to bring out the green, go across from green to the burgundy shades and the purple shades. If you have green-brown hazel eyes and you want to bring the green out, go directly across the color wheel from green and use your warm coppery, burgundy, and purple shades. That will make your hazel eyes pop the most.

The next thing to think about when choosing an eye shadow is skin tone. Depending on the depth of your skin tone, your shade choices can make a significant difference in the intensity of your look. For example, if you have dark ebony skin, you might choose not to wear eye shadows that are too white or light if you find they make you look ashy. Likewise, if you have fair, pale skin, you might choose not to wear dark black eye shadow unless you're going for a very dramatic look.

Last, you might be tempted to match your eye shadow to your clothing, but be warned: it can sometimes make you look washed out. I'm not saying there aren't times when it can work, but if you're ever in doubt, choose a complementary opposite. It will always make you look your best. I recommend choosing eye shadows that work best with your eye color and your features, not your clothes.

These rules apply to eyeliner, too, because it is so close to the eye as well. Of course, black and brown eyeliners work on everyone, but when using colors, follow the same rules as when choosing eye shadows.

blush

The first thing to know about blush is that it's not meant to contour or reshape your face. It's meant to add life and color to your face. That's why the natural flush rule of thumb for choosing a blush color works so well: What color would you flush to if you were to run around the block? You don't want to use a shade of blush any darker than that.

Opposite are some blush samples next to skin tone swatches so you can see a range of shades that work for each category. You'll notice that some of the shades on the ivory/beige side would look too ashy on bronze/ebony skin, and some of the shades on the bronze/ebony side would be too deep and too brown for ivory/beige. Wearing bronze/ebony shades on ivory/beige skin will just make the wearer look dead or tired. Don't try to pull off something that's too dark for your skin tone. You're always better off going with something more colorful versus too dark.

For ivory or beige skin tones, a blush with a soft peach or a warm pink undertone is a great choice. For darker beige or olive skin tones, use a blush with warm undertones and a richness or intensity, so that the color shows up on your skin—tawny shades of dark coral or rich sienna, for example. For bronze/ebony skin tones, choose a blush with a rich, intensely warm undertone, such as bright apricot or a warm brick, to give your skin a natural glow. For more drama, if you have bronze/ebony skin—especially if your skin is deep ebony—you can choose a rich plum blush.

If you're going to have shimmer or sheen to your blush, I personally prefer one with gold shimmer versus silver shimmer. I think the silver shimmer looks too reflective and ashy, which does not work on bronze and ebony skin. A blush with a gold or warm shimmer, however, works well on darker bronze and ebony skin tones, giving the skin a glow and preventing it from looking ashy.

You'll also find that bright pops of color look amazing on your darker skin tones as well. And sometimes there are universal shades that work on all skin tones, such as a nice apricot color.

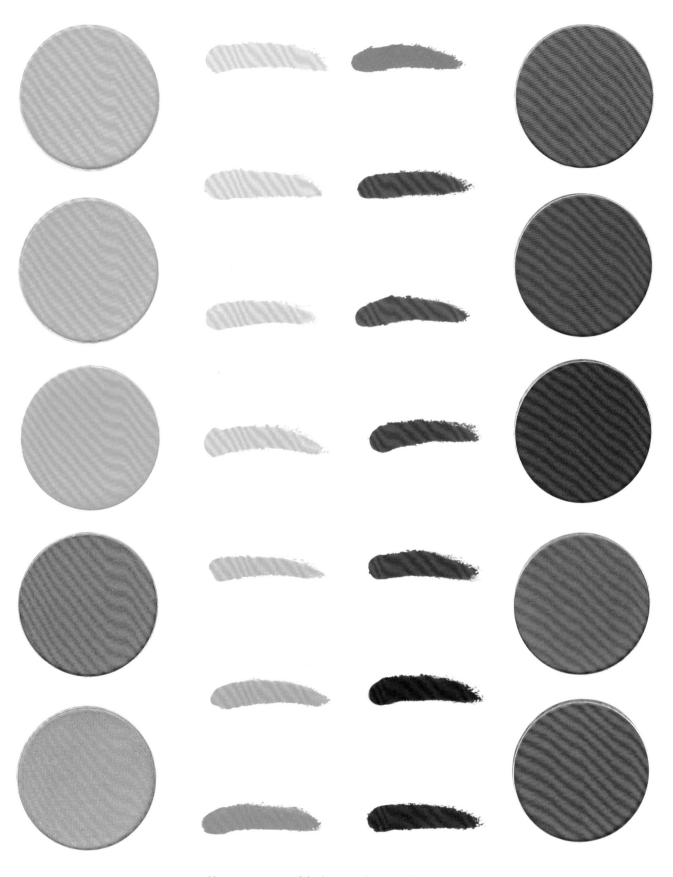

Here are some blush samples next to some skin tone swatches so you can see a range of shades that work for each category.

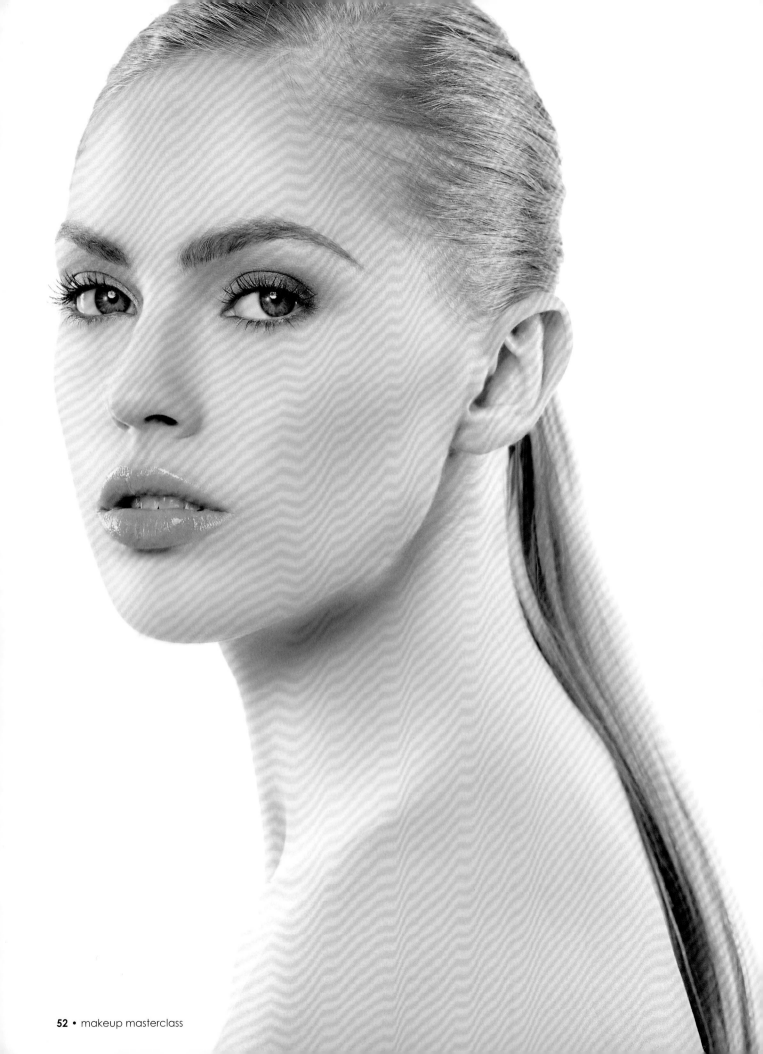

lip color

When it comes to color theory and lipstick, the first question is, how big are your lips? A darker shade of lipstick will make them look smaller, but a lighter shade will make them look fuller. So, if you have thin lips, the last thing you want is a dark shade of lipstick.

Also, if you have ivory or beige skin, the fastest way to age yourself is with a dark lipstick. It's different if you have bronze or ebony skin because the contrast between your skin and the lipstick isn't as high. The fastest way to look younger, especially if you have ivory or beige skin, is using a bright, colorful, warm lipstick; it will add life and color back to your face. If you use a more neutral shade, it could just blend in with your skin. And if you have bronze or ebony skin, a brighter color can brighten your face as well, which helps you look younger.

Your skin tone can influence your color choice too. Consider your skin's undertones. If you have bronze or ebony skin, because it has a brown undertone, brown shades will look very natural on you. If you have ivory or beige skin, because you have no brown in your skin, a brown shade will look too dark and make you look dead.

If your skin is fair, choose a warm pink and a coral or a soft nude color with a soft pink or peachy undertone. For medium complexions, look for shades with a bit more depth. (Remember, the darker your natural lip color, the darker you can go with your lip color choices and have it still look natural.) For medium skin tones, try a deeper rose, a light apricot, or a nude color with a rich apricot undertone. Olive-toned skin is most flattered by rich, tawny shades, soft raisins, and a nude with a rich caramel undertone. Bronze definitely benefits from shades with a bit of brown in them; try a rich raisin, a tawny coffee, or a nude with a dark golden beige undertone. Ebony skin needs richer color choices; try a deep walnut, a rich plum, and a nude with a deep ginger-toned brown (because the skin color is so deep).

If you're not sure what to choose and you want to play it safe, you can always wear something a shade or two darker than your natural lip color. It will give you definition without being too much.

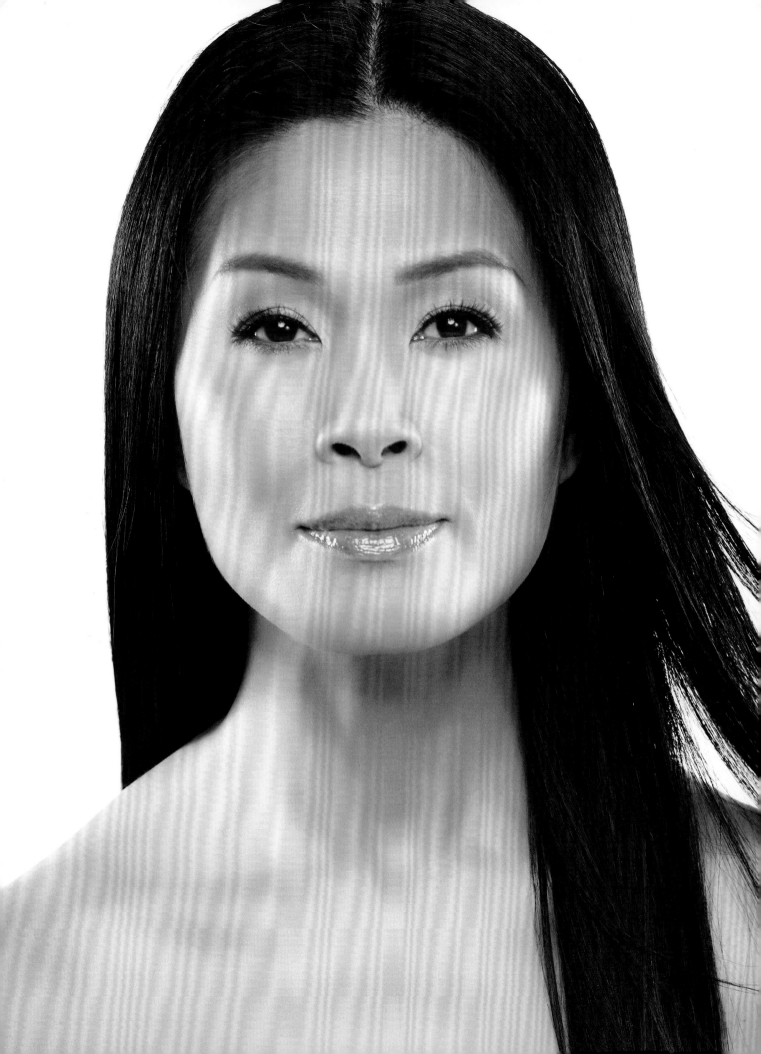

chapter 3

skin deep

Not only will flawless skin make you look your most beautiful, it will also make you look younger. Studies have shown that most people associate discoloration and uneven skin tone with age. In this chapter, we are going to learn how to create the illusion of youthful and flawlessness.

Now let's be realistic: flawless is subjective. I don't want you to expect to look like a cover model when we are finished, but we can certainly make you look your most beautiful. I will show you how to cover all the flaws you don't want to see.

Remember, practice makes perfect. Don't expect to always get it right the first time you try a new technique! Sometimes it is not until the second or third time that it clicks. If you try something and it doesn't work, just wash it off and try again.

how to prepare your skin

The first step to making your skin look its most flawless is preparing and priming it before you apply foundation or concealer. I spend easily as much time prepping the skin for foundation and concealer as I do applying it (sometimes more).

Why prep and prime the face?

- Everything goes on more smoothly.

- Everything stays more flawless longer.

- It helps prevent fine lines from being as visible.

- Your pores will be less visible.

- It helps create a natural glow to the skin.

Here's how to get started.

apply moisturizer

The first step to preparing your skin is to apply moisturizer. Without it, you won't get the flawless application that you deserve. Moisturizer evens out the porosity of your skin, so that everything that follows will adhere evenly and smoothly. No matter what your skin type is, you need to start with moisturizer. Some people with oily skin think they don't need moisturizer, but there is a huge difference between oil and moisture; if you're using the right formula of moisturizer, it will absorb the oil while supplying your skin with all the moisture it needs.

Begin with a freshly washed face and apply your moisturizer while your face is damp, so it goes on more evenly. Take about a quarter-size amount of product, warm it up in your hands, and press it into your face with your palms. The warmth of your hands and pressing it in marries it with your skin, giving it a beautiful glow. Moisturize your entire face and neck. Moisturizer is most effective when it's left to absorb for a few minutes before you apply your makeup. It must be completely dry before you apply anything else.

use eye crème

While you're waiting for the moisturizer to be absorbed, apply eye crème and lip balm so they too have time to absorb before you put anything on top of them. Be very generous with your under-eye crème. Your under-eye area is one of the areas of your body with the fewest moisture glands—and many times the most fine lines—so it can use all the moisture it can get. Moisturizing this area will also help prevent your concealer from creasing.

exfoliate your lips

Keep your lips looking fresh and luscious by exfoliating them. You should exfoliate your lips regularly to keep your lip texture smooth and soft, so your lip color will always go on perfectly. Do this right after you shower. Just apply a generous amount of lip balm and wait a few minutes for it to absorb. Using a soft-bristle toothbrush or a towel, brush your lips vigorously and then apply more lip balm when you're finished.

apply primer

This could be considered an optional step, but for me it's a must. Primer seals in your moisturizer, helps your foundation go on more evenly, and helps it last longer. It sometimes even contains light-reflecting properties that help diminish the appearance of some of your small flaws, so it can help your skin appear fresh-looking all day. It helps prevent foundation and concealer from seeping into fine lines. It also helps prevent your foundation color from altering due to your skin's natural oils because it creates a barrier between those oils and your foundation. Both silicone-based and gel-based formulas do an excellent job. People with oily skin tend to prefer the gel-based formula because of the way the silicone-based formula feels on their skin, but either one can be used on any skin type. Primer is best applied with your fingertips so you can feel where it is going and how much you are applying. Apply it after your moisturizer and eye crème and before your foundation.

foundation

Now that your skin is prepped, it's time to apply foundation. Choosing the right shade of foundation seems to be the hardest thing for most people to do, so don't feel like a failure if you've found it difficult too. Here's what you need to consider when picking your shade and formula.

1. What is the undertone of your skin (olive, yellow, pink, golden orange, or warm brown)?

2. What is the depth level of your skin (pale porcelain all the way to deep ebony)?

3. What is your skin type (oily, dry, combination, sensitive, or normal)?

4. How much coverage do you want (sheer, medium, or full)?

5. What type of finish do you want your foundation to give your skin (matte, satin, dewy, or luminous)?

stripe test

If you have ivory or beige skin tone, conduct the stripe test from your jaw down onto your neck because we want to match your neck. People with ivory or beige skin tend to have redness in their faces, but not in their necks, so it's important to get a true match for the neck. We do not want to apply foundation to your neck—only to your face—so it is imperative that it match your neck and you can stop your application at your jaw. Start by applying stripes of three different foundation shades from your jaw to your neck, making sure to completely blend them. Then, wait a few moments to see if the color shifts or changes as it settles into the skin.

The only way to get an exact shade match for your foundation is to do a stripe test. Here's how:

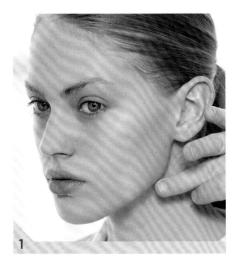

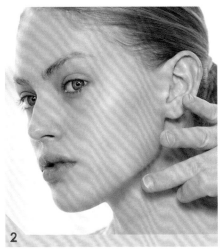

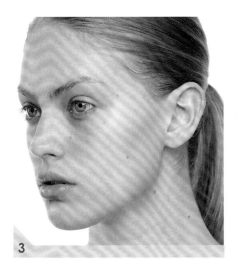

1. Find a spot with natural light.

2. Try multiple shades to make sure you have the perfect match.

3. The shade that matches your neck is the right shade.

If you have bronze or ebony skin tone, conduct the stripe test from your cheek down to your jaw. Many people with these skin tones have multiple shades of skin within their face. (Also, some people with these skin tones have what is called facial masking, lighter skin on the interior of the face and darker skin on the outer edges of the face; if you do, see page 83.)

Stripe testing from your cheek to your jaw will cover any skin tone variations. Start by applying stripes of three different foundation shades from your cheek to your jaw area, making sure to completely blend them. Wait a few moments to see whether the color shifts and let them settle into your skin. Select the one that most closely matches your neck.

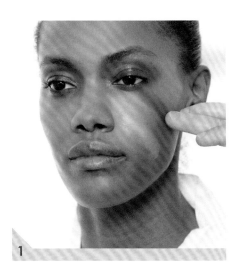

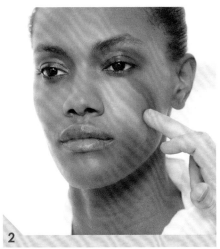

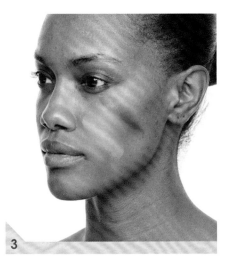

tip: *The best way to keep shine away on oily skin is to use blotting papers to absorb excess oil before you powder. You'll use less powder to eliminate shine.*

Q & A

Whenever I try to get a match for my foundation, the lighting in the store makes it impossible to tell if the shade is correct or not. How can I make sure it matches?

When stripe-testing in a department store, carry a mirror with you so you can walk outside into natural daylight to see which shade is your perfect match. If you are buying foundation at your local drugstore, you obviously can't try the shades on your skin. Still, bring a mirror with you. Take the three shades that most closely match your skin and walk to the nearest window. Hold each bottle close to your face to see which is the closest match. If you are not sure, you could always buy the two that look the closest and mix them to get your perfect shade.

It seems like I can never find the perfect shade! When I compare shades, one always seems a little too light and one a little too dark. Which should I choose?

Choose the slightly darker shade. The lighter shade will only make you look older. Just apply it with a light hand and be careful to blend well along your jawline.

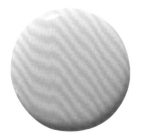 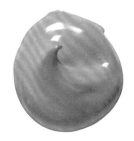 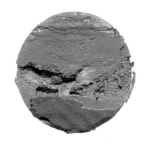

what is your skin's undertone?

A crucial step in creating flawless skin is choosing the right undertone for your foundation. When looking at your face and neck, it is sometimes hard to see your true undertone because of discoloration from the sun and other irritants. But there is another place you can check: the inside of your arm. You wouldn't stripe-test it because it is usually paler than your face and neck, but there's less of a chance for discoloration there, so it's easier for you to see your skin's true undertone.

If you have ivory or beige skin, you will have one of three basic undertones: olive, yellow, or pink. Most people with these skin tones benefit from a foundation with a yellow or olive undertone. A foundation with a yellow or olive undertone will add color and life to the skin, making you look younger.

One of the most common mistakes people with ivory or beige skin make is choosing a foundation with a pink undertone when they don't need it. Even if you have pink in your face, remember that we're matching the neck. The only people who need a pink undertone are people with pink in their faces and necks. Many people think that the pink undertone is adding color to their skin, when it is doing the opposite. It will age you because the pink undertone will make your skin look ashy and old.

If you can't see your undertone, ask yourself: Do I tan easily? If the answer is yes, you will probably need a shade with an olive undertone. If the answer is, "I don't know about easily (I might even burn a little first), but I can get a tan," your skin probably has a yellow undertone. If your answer is, "I always burn rather than tan when I go out in the sun, I couldn't tan if my life depended on it," your skin probably has a pink undertone.

Yellow foundations can visually counteract skin conditions such as rosacea and broken capillaries. If you have one of these conditions or ruddy skin tones, you might feel that foundations with a yellow undertone look too yellow because you're used to seeing all the red in your face. Give it time! Your skin will start to absorb the foundation and work with it better, and your eye will get used to seeing the red neutralized. You'll soon notice a more even, natural, flawless looking skin.

If you have bronze or ebony skin, your undertones are distinct, so match them exactly. They can range from yellow to golden-orange to warm brown. It is also quite possible for you to have multiple shades of skin on your face. Many times, there are lighter areas right above the eyebrows and in the cheek area, with darker areas around the mouth and along the jaw. Don't be afraid to use multiple shades of foundation because by doing so, you can even out your skin. Make sure you apply the correct shade of foundation just to its appropriate shade of skin. If there is a drastic difference between the center of your face and the outer area of your face, see page 83 for more on facial masking.

If you have very deep bronze or ebony skin, you might benefit from brightening (not lightening) your skin. After you have applied your appropriate foundation shade, take a shade of foundation that is one or two shades lighter (in depth) than your natural shade and blend it into the center of your face (the center of your forehead, underneath your eyes, on top of your cheekbones, down the center of your nose, and the tip of your chin). This will give you just a slight, beautiful glow, waking up the appearance of your skin.

What is your skin's depth level?

The depth level of your skin is how light or dark it appears to the naked eye. The paler your skin is, the lighter its depth level is; the darker your skin is, the deeper its depth level is. Match your foundation to your skin's depth level. Choosing a foundation that is too light in depth for your skin can make your face appear lighter and paler than your body, which could age you. Don't choose a shade that is a lot darker than your natural depth level because it will just make your face look darker than your neck and body, which could make your face look muddy and dirty.

What is your skin type?

Using the appropriate formula of foundation for your skin type can make an enormous difference. For example, if your skin type is dry and you do not use a foundation with moisturizers in it, it could accentuate your fine lines (because of lack of moisture). Your dry skin could also absorb the foundation because it's trying to get all the moisture it needs, making it disappear during the day rather than lasting. If your skin type is oily and you do not use a formula with oil absorbers in it (to absorb the excess oil your skin secretes), it could draw attention to facial texture flaws such as large pores and uneven skin texture. If you have combination skin, I would suggest using a foundation with oil absorbers to keep your t-zone (the center of your forehead, nose, cheeks, and chin) from getting too shiny and accentuating textural flaws. If your skin type is normal, your options are much more open.

skin types at a glance

Here are the different skin types, their characteristics, what they need, and which formulas of foundation work best on them.

skin type	characteristics	needs	best foundation
dry	lacks emollients; less elastic; rarely breaks out; feels tight after cleansing; usually small pores; less elasticity; mature skin (very often)	moisturizing foundations; formulas containing emollients and antioxidants; exfoliating regularly	liquid (moisturizing); mousse; tinted moisturizer; bb, cc, and dd creams
normal	neither too oily nor too dry; smooth and even texture; medium to small pores; few to no breakouts; healthy color	pH-balanced products; exfoliating a couple times a week	liquid (all types); crème (all types); mousse; tinted moisturizer; dual-finish; mineral powder; bb, cc, and dd creams
oily	gets shiny fast; usually highly elastic; large pores; can break out often; prone to blackheads; wrinkles less	oil-free products; non-comedogenics; products enriched with oil absorbers; exfoliating regularly	liquid (oil-free); mousse; crème-to-powder; dual-finish; mineral powder
sensitive	sensitive to many products; burns very easily; flushes easily; blotchy (could have dry patches); more susceptible to rosacea; thin and delicate; prone to irritation	hypoallergenic; fragrance-free moisturizing formulas; formulas without chemical sunscreens; best when you can choose formula made for sensitive skin	liquid (water-based); mousse; tinted moisturizer; dual-finish; mineral powder; bb, cc, and dd creams
combination	a mixture of two of the above skin types; usually oily in the t-zone; has a combination of large pores in some areas and smaller pores in other areas; most common combination is oily and normal	may need to use multiple products to appease both areas; exfoliating regularly	liquid (all types); crème (all types); mousse; bb, cc, and dd creams; mineral powder

How much coverage do you want?

This has a little to do with personal preference (do you feel more comfortable with more or less coverage?) and more to do with what you need to look flawless. The sheerer the foundation, the more natural it will look. But you need enough coverage to aid you in covering whatever flaws you do not want to see. Consult chapter 1 (page 12) for a guide to which foundation gives you the right amount of coverage for your skin type. Just remember, sometimes more coverage is about choosing a foundation with more pigment, not adding on more of it.

I have areas of my face that I feel need a little more coverage, but I do not want to wear a foundation with heavier coverage over my entire face. What are my options?

To avoid overly heavy foundation while still getting the coverage you need, you can use two formulas. Apply a sheer formula first and then go back and use a formula that gives you heavier coverage in your trouble spots. This could cut down on the amount of concealer you need, too.

what type of finish do you want your foundation to give your skin?

Your foundation's finish can have an enormous impact on the final look of your skin. Keep in mind that some work better with certain skin types than others. Here are the four basic types:

matte. Matte is a great choice for almost every type of skin, from normal all the way to oily. The only exception is severely dry skin because it could make it look even drier. A matte finish works best on skin with imperfections such as breakouts, scars, and discoloration. (The more matte the skin, the more flawless it will appear because shine just accentuates textural flaws.) A matte finish gives you the best coverage and works well on oily skin because it contains no oils, so it will not increase the shine. However, use a light hand because if you apply it too heavily, it can appear mask-like.

dewy. Dewy works great on dry skin because it adds moisture. It is wonderful for most skin types, except oily skin, on which it can increase the shine and showcase any flaws, such as surface bumps or blemishes. Dewy foundation is not the best choice during summer or in high-humidity areas because it can appear too shiny or greasy instead of just dewy.

satin. The most common foundation finish, satin works on almost all skin types, except for excessively oily skin. It gives the skin a soft, smooth appearance. This finish is extremely kind to skin texture. It isn't as flat as matte, which has no sheen at all, or as shiny as dewy. It makes the skin look young and fresh.

luminous. This works well on almost all skin types. Its light-reflecting properties help hide tiny flaws and lines by reflecting light off the surface of the face. It is also great for giving the skin a healthy glow. Steer clear of this formula if you have oily skin because it could just end up making your face look greasy and oily.

tip: *The more matte your skin, the more flawless it will appear. When in doubt, go matte.*

applying foundation

When applying foundation, you have three basic tools to work with.
All three can give you great application; the best choice for you is the
one you work with best.

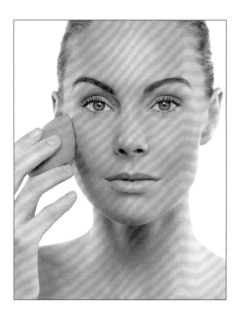

- A sponge is the most sanitary because people are most likely to wash it or throw it away after using it. You must clean it after every use because there is no way to get perfect application from a sponge with dried-up foundation from two days ago in it. The cleaner the tool, the better the application. Sponges also help immeasurably with the blending process. I love sponges. I really feel like I can get the foundation and skin to look like one because I can blend so well. You are in control of your coverage with a sponge. If you stipple (use a patting motion), your sponge will give you more coverage, and if you use it to glide foundation across your face, it will give you less coverage. Always use your sponge damp to help it glide across the skin easier and absorb less product. The higher quality the sponge, the more flawless the application. In the case of sponges, price does matter.

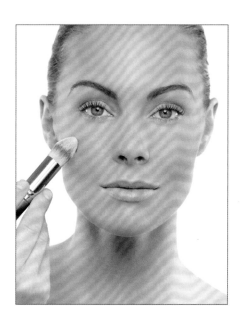

- A brush blends well, so it gives you great coverage. The head of a liquid foundation brush is tapered in its design to promote smooth, even coverage, helping your foundation blend as you apply it. It's great if you want a little extra coverage. It's also excellent for touching up the foundation you've worn all day. If you want to go out in the evening but you don't want to cleanse your face and start over, you can apply more foundation right on top of the product you've had on all day. You can't do that with a sponge or your fingertips. Always wash a liquid foundation brush after every application. Liquid foundation brushes are easy to wash because they are made of synthetic bristles, so they wash more easily and dry faster than natural-bristle brushes. The cleaner the tool, the better the application.

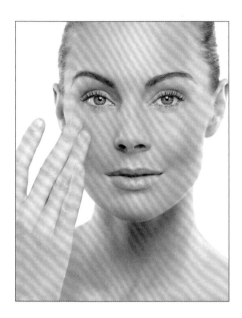

- Don't have a brush or sponge handy? No problem because the third tool is your fingertips. Just make sure to wash your hands after you've applied your moisturizer and treatment products and before you apply your foundation. The residue from the treatment products can compromise the integrity of your foundation and diminish the amount of coverage it provides. Your fingers can give you beautiful, smooth coverage. They're my least favorite tool only because I feel like I can get a better finish with a sponge or a brush. But again, if they're the tool you work best with, they're your perfect application tool.

The center of your face always needs the most coverage, so begin your application there and work outward. You can dip your tool in foundation and apply it directly to your skin, or you can start by dotting foundation on your cheeks, forehead, chin, and nose and then blend it outward. Finish with your final strokes blending downward to make sure all the small facial hairs lie flat.

After application, give the foundation a couple of seconds to dry and then blot it with a tissue to absorb any excess moisture left from the product. Even though powder will absorb excess moisture too, this simple blotting step can really enhance the staying power of your foundation. Be sure to finish with a light dusting of powder. If you have really dry skin, you do not have to powder your entire face: just dust your T-zone (center of forehead, nose, cheeks, and tip of the chin). Many people with dry skin still get shiny T-zones.

tip: *The best way to achieve a natural look is to first go over your entire face with a sheer application of foundation and then go back and apply either another layer of foundation or concealer to any small imperfections.*

concealer

The secret to concealing everything you do not want to see is applying concealer to just the discolored skin. Learn to color within the lines, just like when you learned to color as a child!

There is only one problem with concealer: Designed to stick, it's drier and thicker than foundation. That means it can draw attention to fine lines, especially if you use too much. Choose the right formula for the job. A formula that is too moist can "travel," slipping into creases and fine lines, drawing attention to them. A formula that is too dry is bad for the delicate skin around your eyes and can draw attention to those same flaws. Experiment to find the right formula for you. Consult chapter 1 (page 16) for options.

You also need to choose the right concealer color. When you're just concealing slight discoloration, you should choose the same shade as your foundation or one shade lighter. For extremely dark discoloration, choose a shade that is two levels lighter than your foundation.

If a discoloration is only slight, first try to cover it with a second layer of your foundation before you break out the concealer. Or apply a second foundation, such as stick foundation, that gives more coverage to just the areas that need it. For severe discoloration, you should be more concerned about color correcting than going lighter. For ivory skin, use yellow or a very pale peach for purple or blue discoloration (think dark circles). Don't use a concealer that's too light in depth because it can draw more attention to whatever you are trying to cover. For dark brown spots or redness, use intense yellow. If you have beige skin and want to conceal purple or bluish discoloration, peach will be your best friend. For brown spots and redness, yellow is again what you're looking for. The deeper the beige, the deeper the peach—to almost light orange—you will need to prevent dark circles from going ashy while counteracting the purplish-blue color.

If you have bronze skin, golden orange corrective concealer is your hero. The deeper the discoloration, the more orange and less golden you want. If you have ebony skin, you will want a deep burnt orange corrective concealer on those deep dark spots to help lighten and brighten their depth and bring them up to match the rest of your skin.

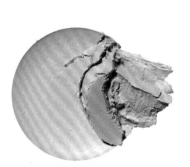

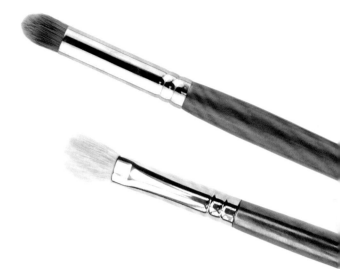

Follow your corrective color concealer with a concealer that matches your natural skin tone to ensure a match. If you're using a concealer that matches your foundation exactly, apply it either before or after your foundation. But if you're using one that is lighter than your foundation or color correcting, apply it first. Stipple (use a patting motion) your foundation over it, making sure everything is blended and concealed to perfection.

Concealers are very different from foundations. They are drier, they're more heavily pigmented, and they "grab" powder differently. So, be careful when you powder over a concealer. It is best to use a lighter shade of powder on any area that you have heavily concealed. If you use the same shade of powder as on the rest of your face, the concealed area will grab the powder and appear darker.

Perhaps you have experienced that proud moment when you concealed a dark spot on your cheek. You used your concealer brush to apply concealer just to the discolored skin and then you stippled all around the edges to blend it in. You looked in the mirror and voilà! No spot. Next, you applied your foundation, stippling it over the area that you concealed to preserve your concealer. Then you powdered to set everything, and suddenly the spot was back. What happened was that the concealer, because of its texture, grabbed the powder that matched your foundation (and your face) and shifted darker. Using a powder that is a shade or two lighter, just on the concealed area, will prevent this from happening.

Let's face it: Very few people have flawless skin. Yet almost everyone is obsessed with perfection! Everything from sun damage to genetics can affect the surface of your complexion, especially as you get older. Fortunately, we can disguise most imperfections. In the pages that follow, let's discuss the techniques you need for specific situations.

dark circles

Concealer can draw attention to fine lines, most often those around the eye. The under-eye area contains fewer oil glands than anywhere else in your body, so it needs plenty of moisture. The moister and suppler you make this area before you apply your concealer, the better the results will be.

Serious dark circles call for serious concealer. Your best option is to use color corrective concealers, which must be applied before your foundation. If you have ivory skin, yellow may be your hero, but for more severe circles, try light peach. If you have severe dark circles on beige skin, you will find that peach correctors will help keep the area from going ashy, especially on deeper beige skin. If you have deeper beige skin, the peach might need to lean a little toward light orange when the dark circle is truly severe. If you have bronze skin, you want an intense golden-orange concealer, but if your dark circles are too severe, you will need it to lean more orange than golden. If you have severe dark circles on ebony skin, you will want a deep orange to help fight that deep brown, almost black, color.

1. Prepare the area underneath your eye: Apply eye crème and let it soak in for a couple of minutes. If the area is really dry, apply an extra layer and let it dry and soak in, too. Be generous with your eye crème because it's next to impossible to "over-moisturize" this area. Just be sure to blot off any excess crème after a few minutes with a sponge or tissue. Using eye crème will help your concealer adhere, and if the skin under your eyes tends to be dry, your concealer won't cake up and draw attention to any fine lines you might have.

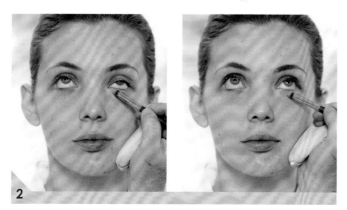

2. Using a brush, apply concealer along the line of demarcation—where the discoloration begins on your skin. Brush the concealer up and over the entire discolored area. You never want to extend the concealer past the line of demarcation onto the skin that you are trying to match. If you do, you will lighten skin that is already the correct color, and you'll be back where you started—with two uneven shades of skin.

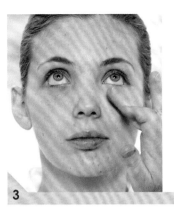

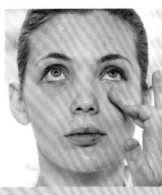

3. With your finger or a stippling brush, stipple the concealer along the line of demarcation. This blends in the texture of the concealer, making it invisible. Be sure to conceal any darkness in the inside corners of your eyes or your eyelids, if necessary.

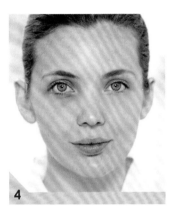

4. Stipple your foundation over the concealed area. You don't want to wipe away what you just concealed. You can see what a difference staying within the lines makes—here with one eye concealed and on not.

5. Finish with a light dusting of powder to set your handiwork.

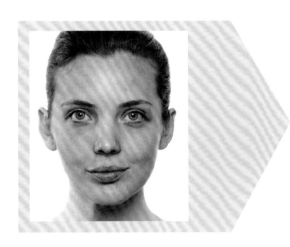

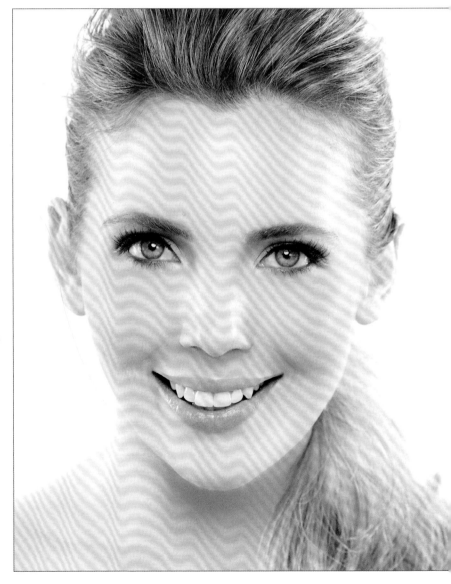

under-eye puffiness

Under-eye puffiness is when the area under your eyes is raised and puffed. The fact that you are usually lit from above accentuates this puffiness because it creates a shadow right underneath the puffy area. You cannot improve the appearance of under-eye puffiness by swiping a light concealer under the eye. That's because anything we lighten will stand out even more. Our goal is to disguise the puffy area, not make it more prominent.

You can outsmart the puffy area by highlighting the area just underneath it, where the puffiness creates a shadow. By highlighting the shadowy area, you will bring it out, making it appear even with the rest of the face, not indented. Because most people look directly at you, your puffiness will appear even with the rest of your skin.

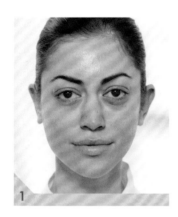

1. Apply your foundation.

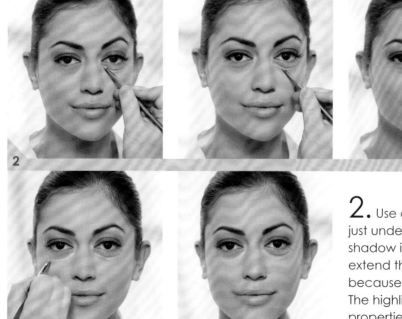

2. Use a highlighting pen (see page 17) just underneath the puffiness, right where the shadow is being created. Make sure not to extend the product up onto the puffy area because it will just make it look puffier. The highlighting pen has light-reflecting properties, making the recessed area come forward so it's even with the rest of the face.

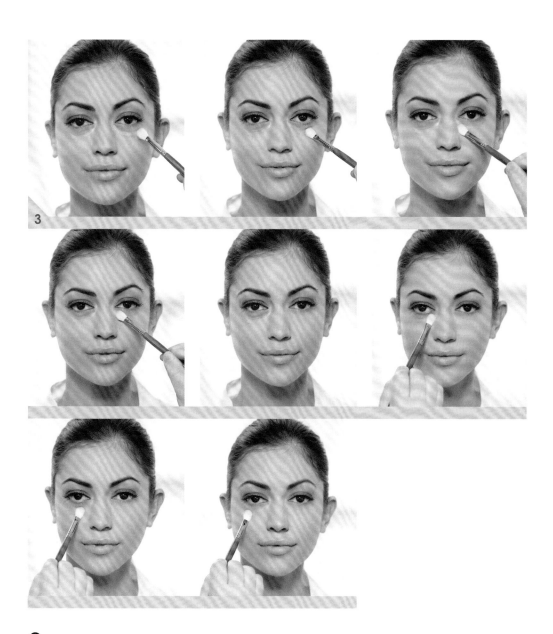

3. With your finger or a stippling brush, stipple all along where you applied the highlighting pen. This will blend in the color and texture, making it invisible.

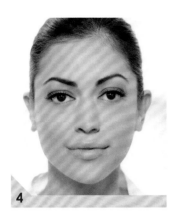

4. Powder lightly and move on with your life.

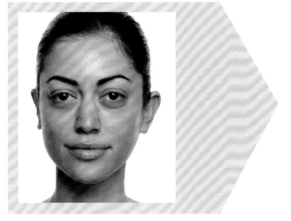

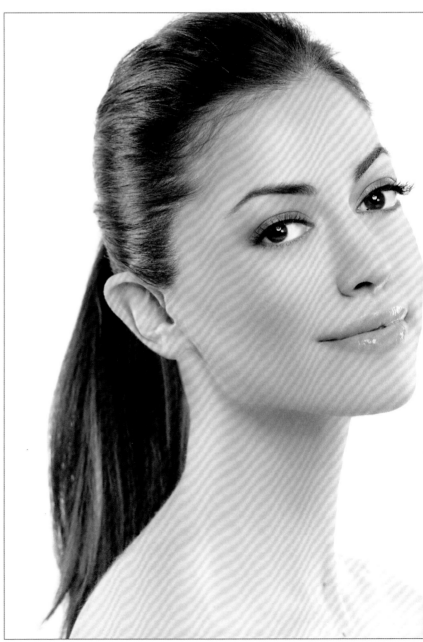

dark circles and puffiness

If you have dark circles *and* puffiness, you will need to take one extra step:

1. Apply concealer to your dark circles first, making sure to only apply it to the discolored skin. Stipple all the edges to blend.

2. Apply your foundation.

3. Apply a highlighting pen right underneath the puffiness, where the shadow is being created (as in step 2 previously).

4. Use your finger or a stippling brush to stipple all along the area where you applied the highlighting pen to blend in the color and texture, making it invisible.

5. Lightly powder and you're done.

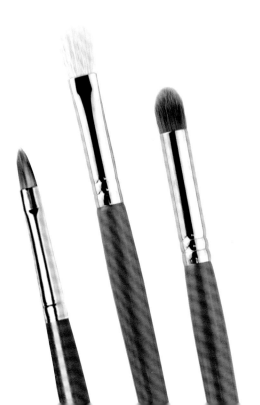

blemishes

To minimize facial blemishes or pimples, use a concealer with a dry texture so it will cling better to the blemish, last throughout the day, and not irritate the skin or initiate more breakouts.

When choosing a concealer, opt for one with a drier texture and a depth level that is not lighter than your foundation. Your concealer should match your skin exactly. A light concealer will only make the blemish seem larger because everything we lighten extends forward.

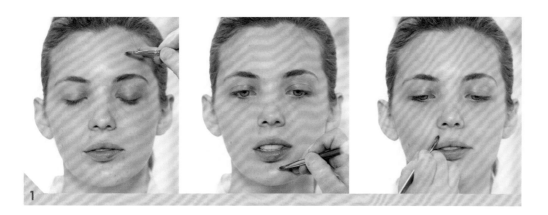

1. Most of your concealing will happen after you apply your foundation for maximum coverage. If there is redness from irritation, start with a light layer of a yellow concealer to neutralize the redness.

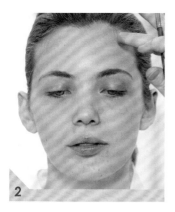

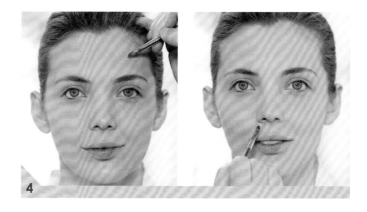

2. With your finger or a stippling brush, stipple to blend in your concealer.

4. Using a brush, apply concealer directly to the blemish.

3. Apply your foundation.

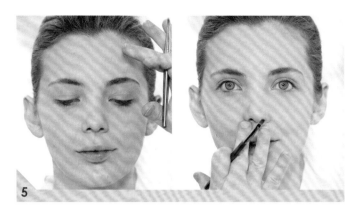
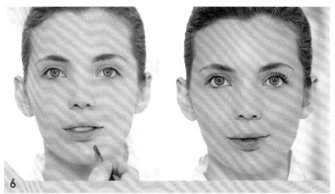

5. With your finger or a stippling brush, stipple to blend the edges all around the blemish into the skin. Stippling blends in the texture of the concealer, making it invisible.

6. Optional: Many times, you might find you want to add a second layer for extra coverage. If you think it would help, apply that second layer and stipple.

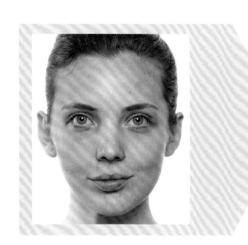

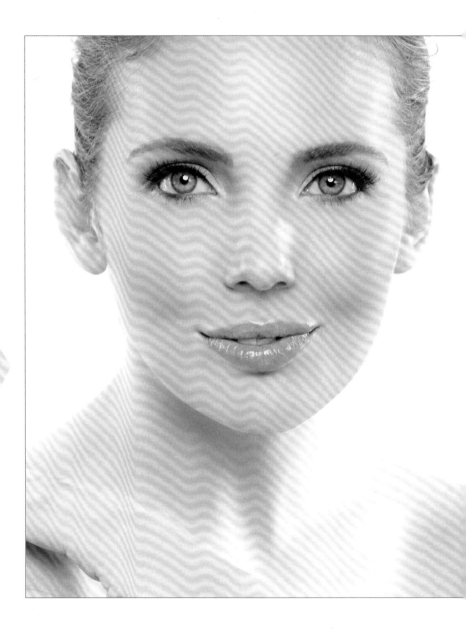

hyperpigmentation or melasma

Hyperpigmentation is a common condition in which patches of skin become darker in color than the normal surrounding skin. This darkening occurs when an excess of melanin, the brown pigment that produces normal skin color, forms deposits in the skin. Hyperpigmentation can affect people of every skin tone. You might have seen it in the form of age spots, which occur due to sun damage. Many women develop them during menopause. These small, darkened patches are usually found on the hands, face, or other areas frequently exposed to the sun.

Melasma spots are similar in appearance to age spots, but are larger areas of darkened skin that appear most often because of hormonal changes. Pregnancy, for example, can trigger an overproduction of melanin that causes "pregnancy masking" (or chloasma) on the face.

If you are prone to hyperpigmentation, stay out of the sun and wear lots of sunblock. Sun exposure just increases the problem. You could have one large spot (more common with pregnancy masking) or multiple small spots. Apply concealer only to the areas that are discolored. If you extend the concealer past the line of demarcation, you will lighten skin that is already the correct color, re-creating multiple shades of skin.

If you have deep brown discoloration on ivory or beige skin, use a yellow pigmented concealer. The deeper the brown and the deeper beige your skin tone, the more your concealer should shift to a dark peach or light orange. If you have bronze or ebony skin tones, use a concealer with a golden orange undertone, all the way into orange depending on how deep the spot is. This will help neutralize the spot color.

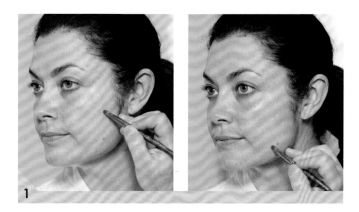

1. Using a brush for precision (unless you have a very large spot, in which case you can use your fingers or a sponge), apply your concealer only to the dark, discolored area. Color within the lines. If there are multiple spots, cover each one separately.

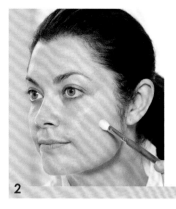 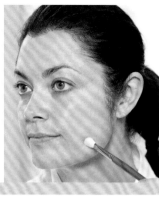

2. Using your finger or a stippling brush, stipple all around the outer edges of every spot that you concealed. This will blend in the texture, making the area look completely natural.

3. Apply your foundation, making sure to stipple it over the areas where you applied your concealer. If you were to wipe your foundation over these areas, you could remove the concealer; stippling prevents that.

4. Finish with a light dusting of powder to set everything and make it last throughout the day.

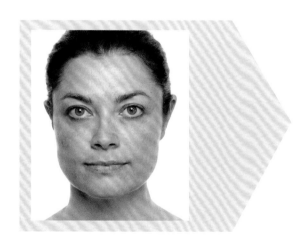

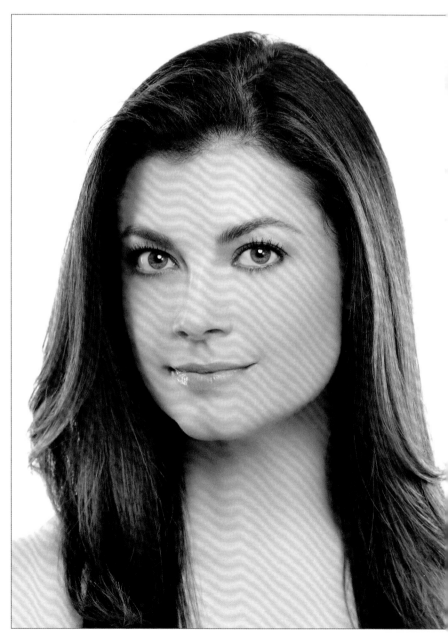

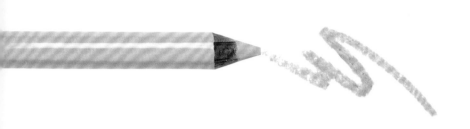

broken capillaries or veins

The trick here is to apply concealer only to the areas of discoloration. Color within the lines. This can be a little difficult with broken capillaries or veins because we must be so exact, but keep practicing and your makeup will get better every day.

A concealer brush will make this process much easier because it is so precise. Or, using a concealer pencil for concealing veins is amazing. You simply draw it right along the vein.

1. Use a concealer brush or pencil to draw a line of concealer right along the broken capillary or vein. You can't just conceal the general area; you must apply it only to the vein. If you extended the concealer past the edges of the vein or broken capillary, it will lighten the skin you're trying to match, disguising nothing.

2. Using the tip of your finger or a stippling brush, stipple all along where you applied your concealer. This will blend in the texture of your concealer and make it look completely natural.

3. Next apply your foundation. As with any time you apply foundation over concealer, stipple your foundation over the concealed area.

4. Powder to set everything and help it last all day.

rosacea

Rosacea is an area of redness on the skin, usually a general area of redness with some darker red spots. It most commonly occurs in the cheek area and across the nose, as well as the chin and sometimes the forehead. A lot of women start to develop slight cases after they start having the hormonal changes of menopause. And other people have rosacea their whole lives.

1. Make sure the rosacea area is as smooth and moist as possible. Most times it is dry and flaky and needs to be exfoliated. But you cannot exfoliate it with normal exfoliators, which would just irritate the area. Do it with moisturizer: Slather a heavy moisturizer over the entire area and let it sit for about 5 minutes. Then with a damp nubby washcloth, lightly rub in a circular motion. The moisturizer will have softened the dead dry skin and the washcloth will roll it right off. Now cleanse and moisturize like normal, and the area will be nice and smooth.

2. To counteract the redness of rosacea, you will need a yellow-based concealer. Apply a thin layer of concealer to the entire area and to all areas that are red. This thin layer will get rid of the general area of redness, but you will probably be left with a few darker areas still showing through.

3. Using the same concealer, go back and apply another layer to the darker areas that are still showing through (but only to the spots that are still visible). By covering in two steps, you do not have a thick layer of concealer over a large area of your face, so your skin looks more natural.

4. Stipple all around the outer edges of the area you concealed to blend in the texture.

5. Apply your foundation, making sure to stipple rather than wipe your foundation over the areas you just concealed. If you were to wipe on the foundation, it could remove the product where you just concealed.

6. Finish with a light dusting of powder.

Most people, after they conceal their rosacea, do not want to wear blush. They just got rid of the excess color in their cheeks, and the last thing they want to do is add some back. If you do want color back in this area, choose something very natural. An excellent choice is just a little bronzer for color rather than blush.

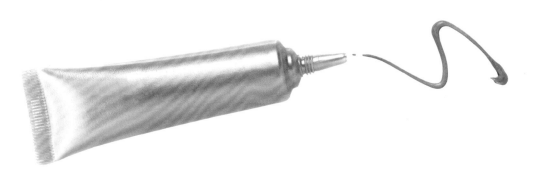

vitiligo or hypopigmentation

Vitiligo (also called hypopigmentation or leukoderma) is a chronic skin condition that causes loss of pigment, resulting in irregular pale patches of skin. You're dealing with light spots (spots with no pigment) on the skin to conceal. As with dark spots, the trick is to color within the lines when applying your concealer because if the concealer extends past the line of demarcation, you will once again have multiple shades of skin.

What makes vitiligo so different is that instead of using a concealer to lighten a spot, we actually need one to deepen a spot. The deeper your skin tone is, the deeper your concealer will need to be. If you have beige skin, you will probably need a shade of concealer only one to two levels darker than your natural skin. But if you have bronze or ebony skin, you will probably need a shade two to three levels darker than your natural skin tone.

1. Using a brush for precision (unless it is a large spot, in which case you can use your fingers or a sponge), apply your concealer only to the light discolored area. If there are multiple spots, cover each one separately.

2. Using your finger or a stippling brush, stipple all around the outer edges of every spot that you concealed. This will blend in the texture, making the skin look completely natural.

3. Apply your foundation, making sure to stipple it over the areas on which you applied your concealer. If you were to wipe your foundation over these areas, you could remove the concealer; stippling on foundation will prevent this.

4. Finish with a light dusting of powder to set everything and make it last throughout the day.

facial masking

Facial masking is a condition that sometimes affects people with bronze or ebony skin tones. It means your skin has a natural "mask," a tendency to be darker around the outer edges of your face and lighter on the interior. It will take two shades of foundation or concealer to correct this.

Correcting facial masking is different from any other concealing that you will do because when you are dealing with facial masking, there are actually three shades of skin to consider: the light area in the center of your face; the much darker area all around the outer perimeter of your face (your forehead, jawline, and around your mouth); and the color of your neck and body, which is usually lighter than the outer edges of your face, but darker than the center.

1. Conduct a stripe test from your cheek down to your jaw to determine the two foundation or concealer shades you will need to create a more even complexion (see pages 58 and 59). One shade will brighten the darker areas and one will deepen the lighter areas. You can't use just one shade because there is no way one shade can lighten the darker area to match the lighter area; you also don't want to deepen the lighter area to match the dark (because remember, the darker area is darker than your neck and body). The goal of your stripe test is to find the two shades that, when applied to the opposite areas of your skin, meet in the middle (or make each area match the other). You want to slightly lighten the dark area and slightly deepen the light area.

2. Apply the lighter shade of foundation to just the darker areas on your face.

3. Apply the darker shade of foundation to just the lighter areas on your face. Applying the appropriate shade of foundation to the correct shade of skin will correct your skin tone and make your skin look even and flawless.

4. You will have to wait until you have finished evening out your skin tone to decide what powder shade you will need. When you have, apply powder to set your makeup.

scars

Scars are especially tricky to conceal, because a scar is an area of skin that has no pores, and pores are what makeup clings to on the skin. Foundation just slips right off. You will need a special concealer—one that has a much drier texture than, for example, one you would use under your eyes—to get it to adhere to the scar.

If you have a concealer that is drier in texture and designed to conceal scars, here's how to use it:

1. With a concealer brush, apply your concealer directly to the scar (and only to the scar).

2. With your finger or a stippling brush, stipple all around and along the edges of the area where you applied your concealer. This will blend in the texture of your concealer and make it invisible.

3. As you are applying your foundation, when you reach the area you just concealed, stipple the foundation over your scar. Don't wipe it on—you don't want to expose the scars you just concealed.

4. Lightly powder to set your makeup so it will last all day.

If you do not want to invest in multiple concealers, you can adjust your normal concealer so that it will adhere to the scar:

1. Lightly moisturize the scarred area.

2. Powder the scar with a tiny bit of loose powder. The moisturizer should give the powder something to cling to.

3. With a concealer brush, apply your concealer directly to the scar (and only to the scar). The concealer and powder will mix together, creating a drier texture so it can adhere to the scar.

4. With your finger or a stippling brush, stipple all around and along the edges of the area on which you applied your concealer. This will blend in the texture of your concealer and make it invisible.

5. As you are applying your foundation, when you reach the area you just concealed, stipple it over your scar. Don't wipe it on, or it could remove the concealer-powder blend.

6. Powder lightly to set your makeup so that it will last all day.

For acne scars, which create texture variation in your skin, keep everything as matte as possible. You want to make sure you keep all the oils and shine away all day, so blot often and use loose powder to matte the skin.

Keep the finish of your color products in mind as well: Any sparkle or shimmer in your blush or bronzer, for example, will make your skin look shiny, accentuating your textural flaws. The more matte the skin, the more flawless it will appear.

Finally, resist the temptation to try to fill in the "valleys" by applying too much foundation and concealer. Trying to cover up the textural flaws with thick, heavy layers of concealer and foundation will just make your skin look caked. A nice, smooth matte layer will make you look fresher and will make your skin look its most flawless.

tattoos

When you are covering a tattoo, it is probably not going to be where you will also be applying foundation. That is, it will likely be on your neck, wrist, ankle, or the like—not your face. Because you won't be applying any foundation over the tattoo, you need to make sure you have an absolutely perfect color match. You also need a product that is drier in texture than foundation so it sticks better and stays put all day.

Your tattoo is likely to be much darker than the skin it is on (most tattoos have purplish-blue, almost black borders). If that's the case, your goal is to over-lighten the tattoo and then bring it back down to the color of the skin.

You will need three different concealer colors to accomplish a natural looking cover. The first is a peachy color for ivory skin, a deep peach for beige skin, an even deeper peach, almost light orange, for dark beige skin, an orange for bronze skin, or a deep burnt orange for ebony skin. The second is a light concealer (lighter than your skin tone), and the third is an exact skin match.

(tattoos continued)

1. Color within the lines as much as possible! Using a concealer brush and your color-correcting concealer, color directly over the tattoo. Build the color; start with less and add layers rather than putting too much on initially.

2. Stipple the first layer with your finger or a stippling brush.

3. With a brush, sponge, or powder puff, apply a thin layer of a transparent setting powder—one designed specifically for applications such as this.

4. Using a concealer brush, apply another layer of your color-correcting concealer directly over the tattoo, again trying to stay within the lines.

5. Stipple with either a stippling brush or a foundation brush, so you don't remove too much product.

6. Stipple over the entire tattoo area with a foundation brush or sponge and the lighter skin tone concealer.

7. Stipple again with a stippling brush or sponge.

8. Change to the natural skin tone concealer and stipple over the entire tattoo area of the tattoo with a foundation brush or sponge.

9. Finish with a final dusting of powder to set the area.

tip: *Don't be afraid to add more translucent powder between layers and stipple over the area again with more product. This will help the product stick and stay put.*

beards

The trick to covering a five o'clock shadow is using the right color-correcting concealer and not necessarily a certain amount of concealer. Due to the darkness and tone of the shadow, you will need something in the peachy to orange family. If you have ivory skin, use a light peach. If you have beige skin, use a darker peachy color. If you have dark beige skin, use a deep peach going into an almost light orange. If you have bronze skin, you will need orange. And if you have ebony skin, you will need a deep burnt orange. These shades will counteract the dark brown to almost black shadow created from the shadow.

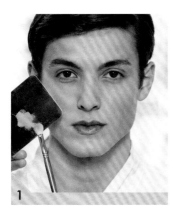

1. Using a foundation brush, concealer brush, or sponge, depending on how large the area you're covering is, apply your color-correcting concealer. Stay within the lines (that is, only apply concealer to the shadowed area).

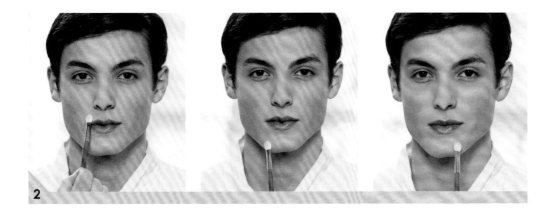

2. With your finger, a stippling brush, or a sponge, stipple all around the edges to blend in the concealer and the texture.

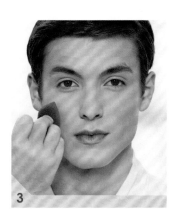

3. Apply foundation normally (see page 66), except when you get to the beard area, stipple it so you don't remove any of the concealer and you get maximum coverage.

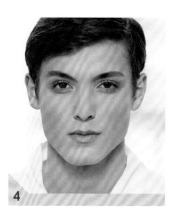

4. Powder to set your foundation. Consider using a no-color transparent setting powder on your beard so it doesn't darken the concealed area.

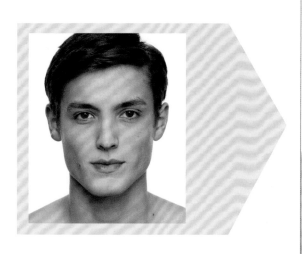

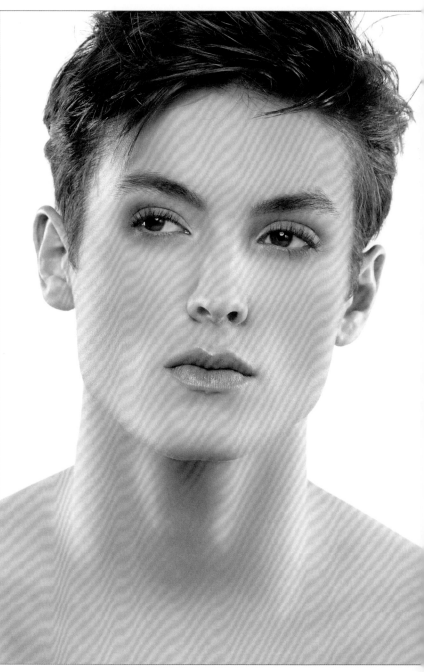

powder

Powder sets your foundation, polishes your look, and adds a smooth, velvety softness to your skin. Because loose powder contains more oil absorbers than pressed powder, I prefer to use it to set the foundation. You can always use pressed powder for touch-ups throughout the day because it is fast and easy to carry.

Choose a shade of powder that matches your foundation. The powder will reinforce everything you have applied (foundation, concealer, highlighting pen). You can also use a translucent powder, which is fine for paler skin tones. It is less opaque than other powders, but it is not colorless, and it can often appear unnatural and ashy on dark beige, olive, bronze, and ebony skin tones. The one time translucent powder is helpful is when powdering areas that have been heavily concealed on ivory or beige (but never bronze or ebony) skin.

There are several ways to apply both types of powder:

- A brush is the easiest and most commonly used tool. It will give you a nice light powder coverage. It is great for blending, but you must be careful not to over-blend and brush off what you apply. For best results, apply a little bit of powder at a time with a brush, instead of applying it all at once, to ensure smooth, even coverage. If you are using loose powder, simply dip your brush in powder and then tap it in the palm of your hand (or the top of the powder jar) to remove the excess. Apply what's left on the brush to your face. Then use your brush to pick up the powder that's left in your palm or the top of the jar and finish applying it to your face.

- A powder puff offers the most coverage. Press your puff into the powder, tap the excess off in the palm of your hand, and then roll what is left on the puff onto your skin. Then grab the leftover powder in your palm with the puff and finish applying it to your face. Pushing it into the skin makes your foundation and powder appear as one with your skin; it looks more natural while giving you complete coverage. To finish, lightly sweep your face with a brush, using gentle downward strokes to remove any excess powder.

- A fingertip works well for the lightest powder application. It's a terrific way to powder underneath the eyes, especially when you don't want to draw attention to fine lines. Just dip your finger in loose powder. Rub it in the palm of your hand to brush off the excess and then trace your finger over the area underneath your eyes to set your concealer.

- A sponge works well for tight areas and is great for spot powdering. It will give you maximum coverage like a puff does.

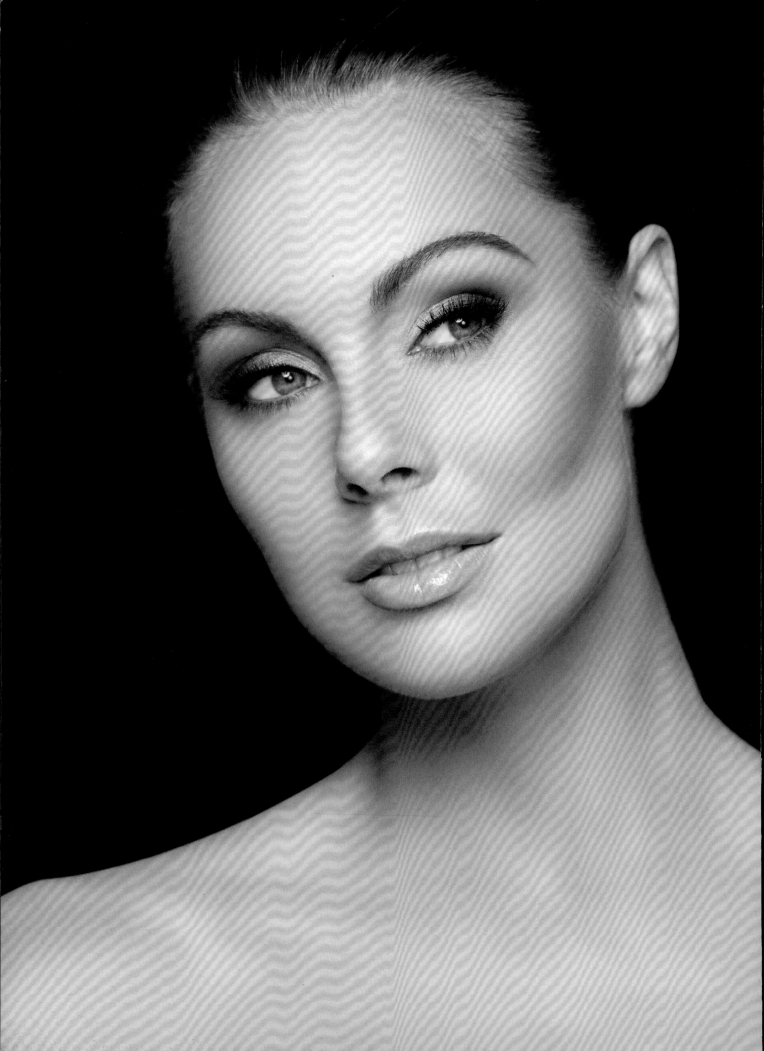

chapter 4

face map

Makeup can be transformative. And no makeup technique you master will have a bigger impact on that transformation than combining highlighting and contouring. It's been in the media a lot lately, but makeup artists have always used it. I've practiced it since the beginning of my career, and mastering it has truly set me apart as an artist.

It's the makeup artist's version of an optical illusion. You can use it to change the appearance of your face shape: Everything you highlight (or lighten) comes forward visually, and everything you contour (or darken) moves into the background.

The face shape that's considered the most perfect is oval. By highlighting and contouring, you can make your face appear more oval, thinner, or more sculpted. You'll highlight the areas of your face you want to see (the oval area) and contour the areas you don't.

This technique also adds color, warmth, and light. The subtle effect gives your skin an incredible glow. This is an optional step, but once you experience the benefits, you'll love it.

choose the right shades: ivory/beige skin

First, select three shades of foundation and/or powder in three different depth levels. It works best if the three shade are all the same texture, because they will blend more easily.

1. The first color, your true foundation color, should match your skin exactly.

2. The second color, your highlight color, should be at least one level lighter than the first, preferably with the same undertone.

3. The third shade, your contour color, should be at least one level darker than your first, preferably with the same undertone.

The more dramatic you want your result to be, the more dramatic the contrast between the three shades' depth levels should be. For noticeable contouring on ivory or beige skin, use a contour shade that is two to three levels darker than your natural shade. The more dramatic your choices, the more thoroughly you will have to blend the shades together.

How do you know where to place what shades? It's simple! Picture an oval on your face, as wide as your eye sockets and extending from the tip of your forehead to the tip of your chin.

Now it's simply a matter of lightening all the high points inside the oval and contouring or darkening everything outside the oval.

In the images opposite and on page 100, I have over-exaggerated what to highlight and what to contour. The light color indicates where to highlight: the center of your forehead, down the center of your nose (if you want to visually narrow it), under your eyes, on top of your cheekbones, the tip of your chin, and the top of the bow of the lips (to make them look fuller). The dark color indicates where to contour: your temples, all along your cheekbones (some would say under, but this could widen the appearance of your face), along the sides of your nose up into your crease, just under the lower lip to create a shadow (to make it look fuller), and along your jawline to define it.

If you have ivory or beige skin, you will contour your face more than you highlight. With very fair skin, you want to avoid appearing washed out. Contouring will give you the most dramatic change. For bronze or ebony skin, you will highlight your skin more than contour. Contouring may get somewhat lost if you have darker bronze or ebony skin tones, while highlighting will brighten and bring life to your skin.

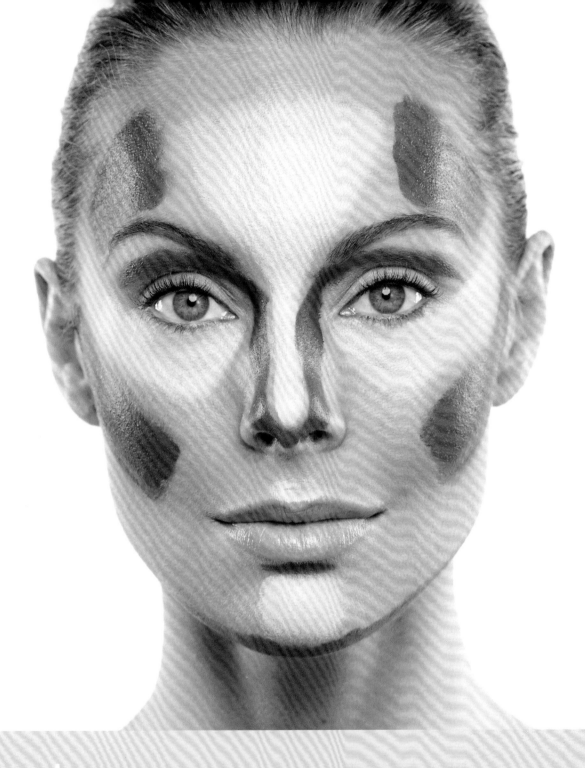

benefits of highlighting and contouring

- Your face will have a youthful glow and color.

- Lifting the eyes (when you contour your temples) will make you look younger.

- Your face shape will be narrowed or broadened, as you desire.

- Your jaw will be defined.

- Your lips will look fuller.

- Your nose will look thinner, if you want it to.

- Your cheekbones will be lifted.

how to sculpt your face

ivory/beige skin tone

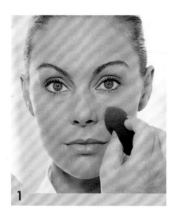

1. Apply your first, or true, foundation color over your entire face. Then visualize an oval on your face. The width of the oval is from the outside of one eye socket to the outside of the other; the height of your oval extends from the tip of your forehead to the tip of your chin.

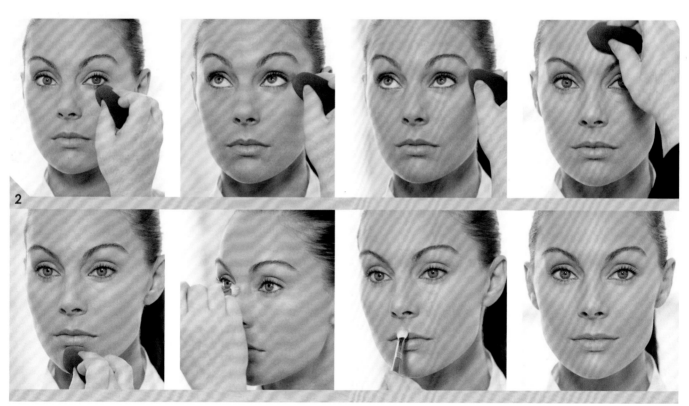

2. Apply your second, or highlight, foundation color to the high points inside the oval, including under your eyes, on top of your cheekbones, the center of your forehead, and the tip of your chin. Use brush #59 (for more control) down the center of your nose (if you want to visually narrow it) and the top of the bow of the lips (to make them look fuller).

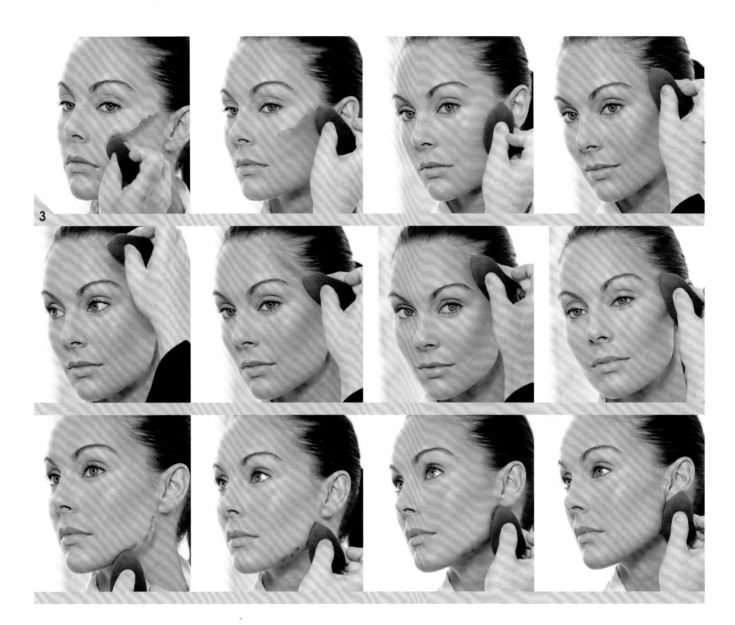

3. Apply your darkest, or contour, shade to the areas outside the oval, including all along your cheekbones, your temples, and along your jaw-line. By deepening the outside areas, you are visually helping those areas recede, making your face appear more narrow and oval.

tip: *If you're short of time and want a similar but less dramatic effect, contour with a matte bronzer after you apply your foundation.*

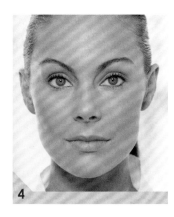

4. Blend everything well. The secret to making your highlights and contours look appearing is all in the blending.

5. Apply powder in a shade that matches your natural skin tone. It won't negate all your work; instead it will set everything beautifully.

For even more dramatic results, finish with three shades of powder: one that matches your true foundation shade, one that matches your highlight shade, and a darker or matte bronzing powder to match your contour shade. This will reinforce your work and give you a beautifully sculpted, three-dimensional effect that will make any face shape appear more oval and add that ever-so-important glow.

Your neck is likely paler than your face, so extend your matte bronzer down onto your neck; don't just stop at your jawline. It will help your entire face and neck match your décolletage.

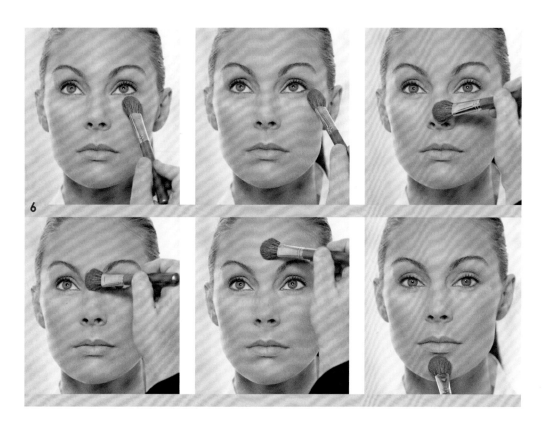

6. Using brush #76 and a no-shimmer translucent highlight powder, set your highlight under your eyes and on top of your cheekbones, up the center of the nose, the center of the forehead, and the tip of the chin. Be generous but mindful that with age and thinner skin, more powder draws attention to fine lines. Brush off excess highlight powder.

tip: *Shimmer highlight powder can draw attention to skin texture and flaws. Choose no-shimmer to avoid this issue.*

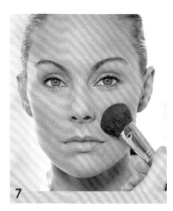

7. Using powder brush #73, powder the rest of your face with a powder that matches your exact foundation.

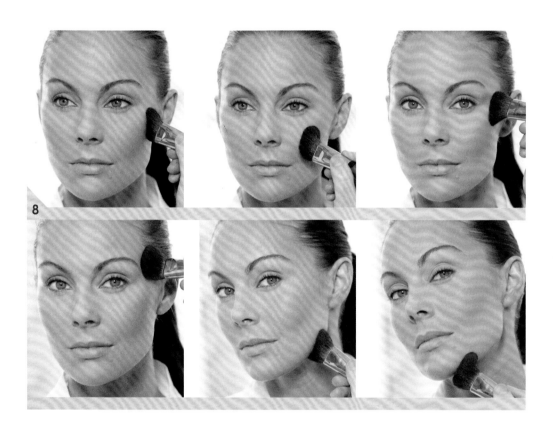

8. With bronzing brush #73, reinforce your contour using a matte bronzer (never shimmer, which will expand the face shape, not contour it). Begin at the back of your cheekbone and sweep it forward to the apple of your cheek. Then take the brush back toward your ear. This lays the color in place. Next, move your brush in the opposite direction (up and down) to blend well. Don't forget to add a little at the temples to help add shape and a glow. Sweep the bronzing powder up around the temples and eye socket. Finish by applying it along your jawline.

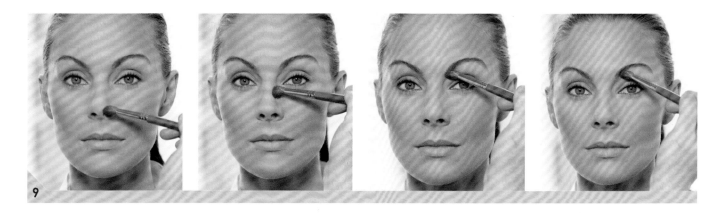

9. Using brush #11 and matte bronzing powder, sweep your brush up along the sides of your nose up into the beginning of your brow and crease. Apply across the tip of your nose, blending the edges well.

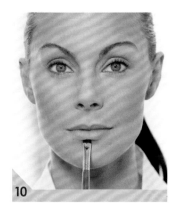

10. With brush #38 and matte bronzing powder, define just below your lower lip to create a deeper shadow and give the illusion of a fuller lip.

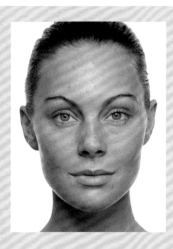

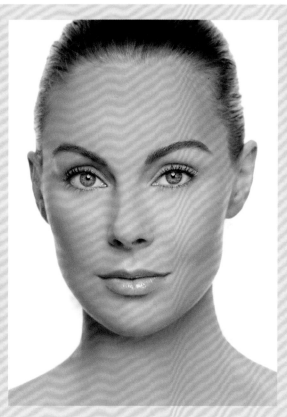

You can see how we have added shape, color, and a beautiful glow to her face. Highlighting and contouring does worlds of good for the overall appearance of the skin and face.

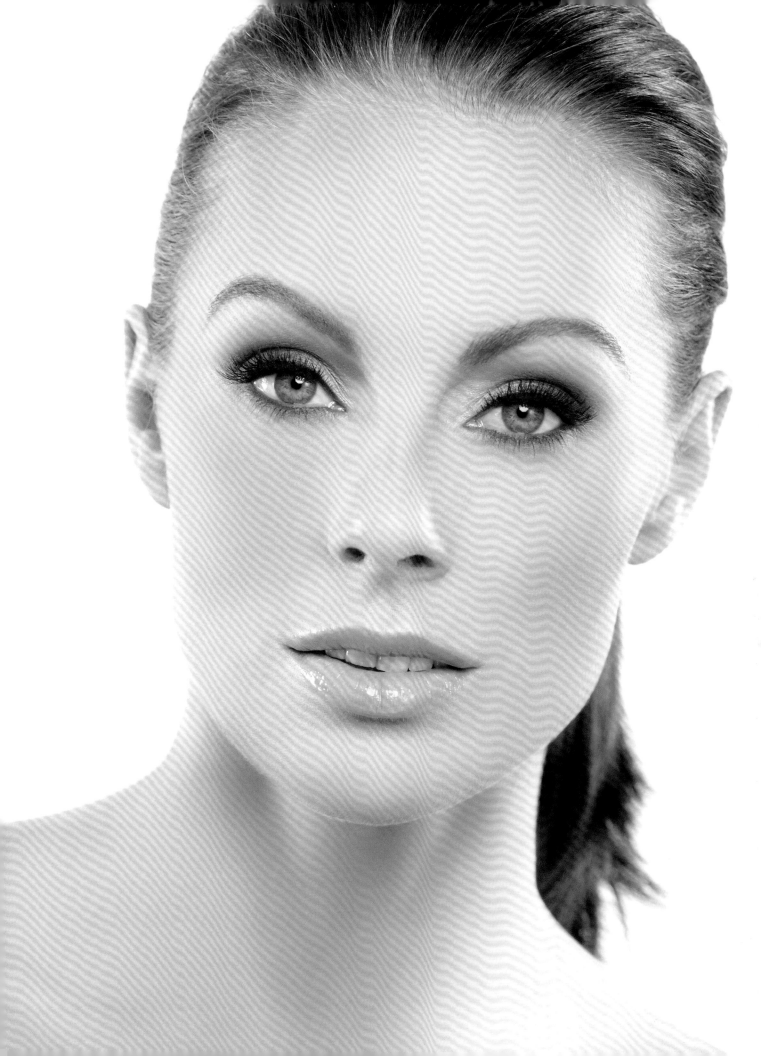

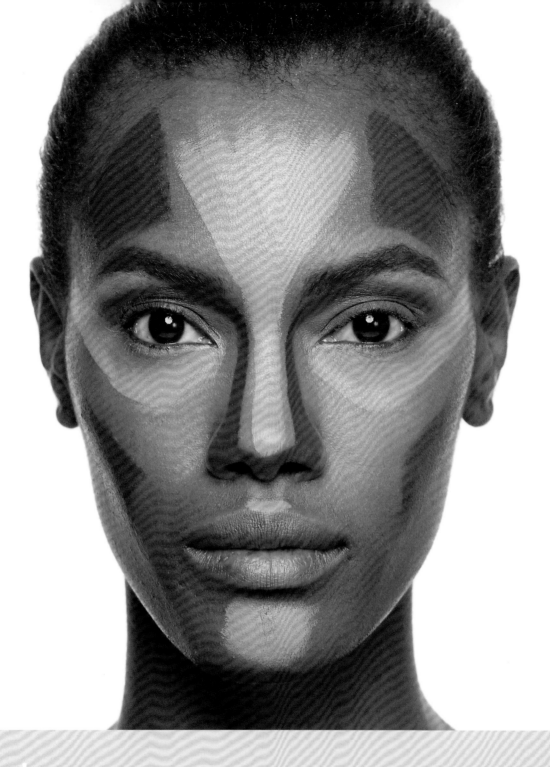

benefits of highlighting and contouring

- Your face will have a youthful glow and color.

- Lifting the eyes (when you contour your temples) will make you look younger.

- Your face shape will be narrowed or broadened, as you desire.

- Your jaw will be defined.

- Your lips will look fuller.

- Your nose will look thinner, if you want it to.

- Your cheekbones will be lifted.

choose the right shades: bronze/ebony skin

First, select three shades of foundation and/or powder in three different depth levels. It works best if the three shade are all the same texture, because they will blend more easily.

1. The first color, your true foundation color, should match your skin exactly.

2. The second color, your highlight color, should be at least one level lighter than the first, preferably with the same undertone.

3. The third shade, your contour color, should be at least one level darker than your first, preferably with the same undertone.

The more dramatic you want your result to be, the more dramatic the contrast between the three shades' depth levels should be. To create contrast on bronze and ebony skin, choose a highlight shade that is two to three levels lighter than your natural shade. The more dramatic your choices, the more thoroughly you will have to blend the shades together.

How do you know where to place what shades? It's simple! Picture an oval on your face, as wide as your eye sockets and extending from the tip of your forehead to the tip of your chin.

Now it's simply a matter of lightening all the high points inside the oval and contouring or darkening everything outside the oval.

In the images opposite and shown on page 92, I have over-exaggerated what to highlight and what to contour. The light color indicates where to highlight: the center of your forehead, down the center of your nose (if you want to visually narrow it), under your eyes, on top of your cheek-bones, the tip of your chin, and the top of the bow of the lips (to make them look fuller). The dark color indicates where to contour: your temples, all along your cheekbones (some would say under, but this could widen the appearance of your face), along the sides of your nose up into your crease, just under the lower lip to create a shadow (to make it look fuller), and along your jawline to define it.

If you have ivory or beige skin, you will contour your face more than you highlight. With very fair skin, you want to avoid appearing washed out. Contouring will give you the most dramatic change. For bronze or ebony skin, you will highlight your skin more than contour. Contouring may get somewhat lost if you have darker bronze or ebony skin tones, while high-lighting will brighten and bring life to your skin.

bronze/ebony skin tone

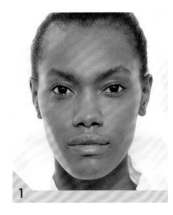

1. Apply your first, or true, foundation color over your entire face. Then, visualize an oval on your face.

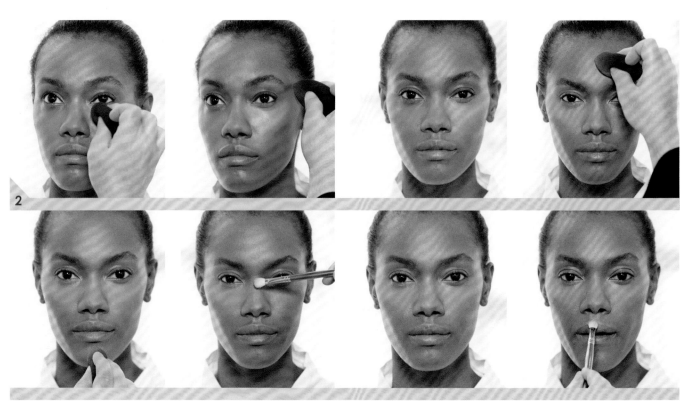

2. Apply your second, or highlight, foundation color to the high points inside the oval, including under your eyes, on top of your cheekbones, the center of your forehead, and on the tip of your chin. Use brush #59 (for more control) down the center of your nose (if you want to visually narrow it) and the top of the bow of the lips (to make them look fuller).

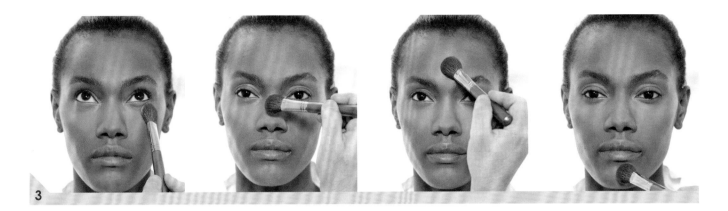

3. Using brush #76 and a no-shimmer translucent highlight powder, set your highlight under your eyes and on top of your cheekbones, up the center of the nose, the center of the forehead, and the tip of the chin.

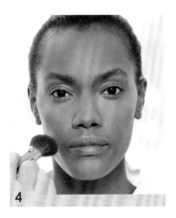

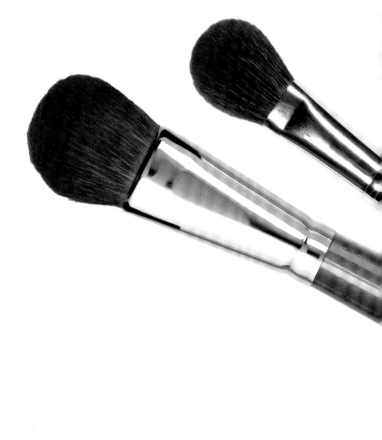

4. With powder brush #73, powder the rest of your face with a powder that matches your foundation exactly.

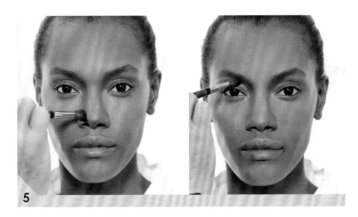

5. Using brush #11 and matte bronzing powder, sweep your brush up along the sides of your nose up into the beginning of your brow and crease. Apply across the tip of your nose, blending the edges well.

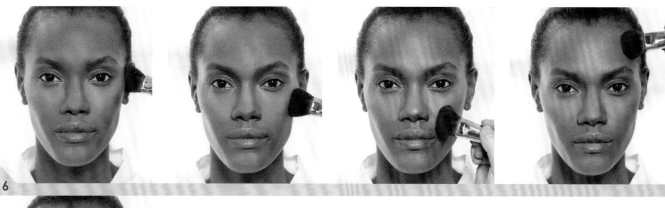

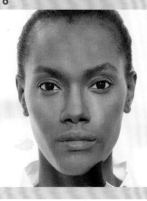

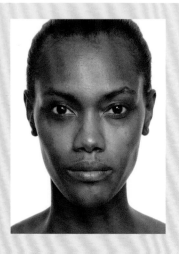

6. With bronzing brush #73, define your contour areas using a matte bronzer (I find one with a hint of raisin tone in it works best). Begin at the back of your cheekbone and sweep it forward to the apple of your cheek. Then take the brush back toward your ear. This lays the color in place. Next, move your brush in the opposite direction (up and down) to blend well. Don't forget to add a little at the temples to help add shape and a glow. Sweep the bronzing powder up around the temples and eye socket. Finish by applying it along your jawline.

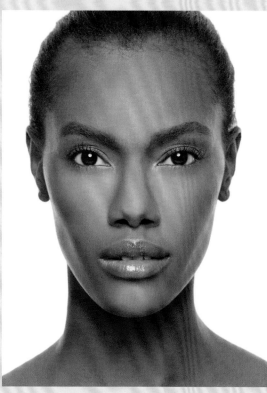

By highlighting her skin tone, it looks as if you almost turned the light on inside her face. It makes such a difference.

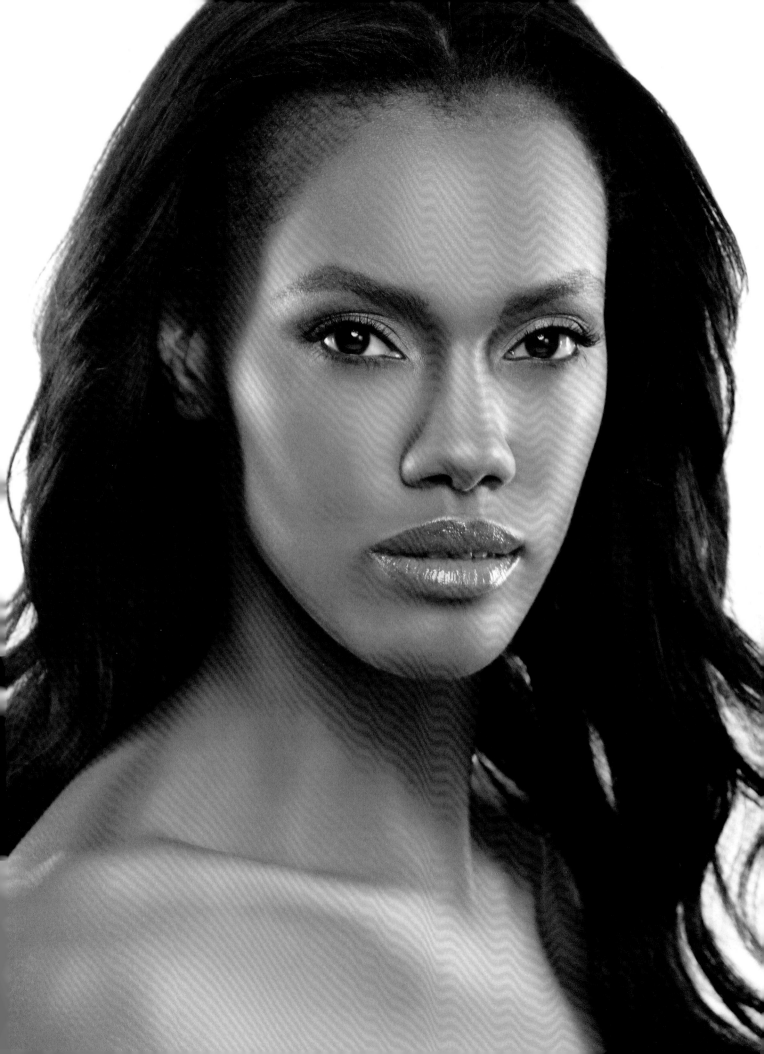

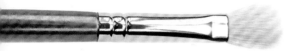

ivory/beige skin tone

1. Apply your first, or true, foundation color over your entire face. Then visualize an oval on your face.

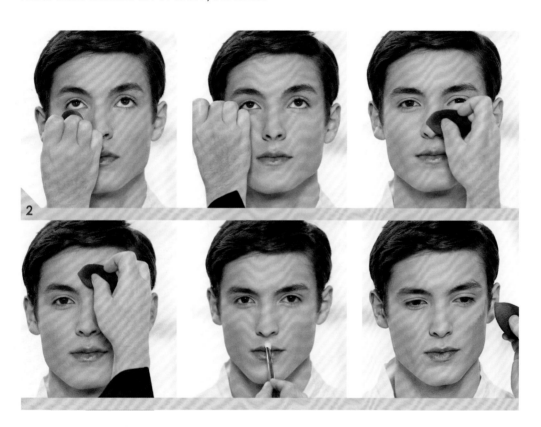

2. Apply your second, or highlight, foundation color to the high points inside the oval, including under your eyes, on top of your cheekbones, the center of your forehead, and the tip of your chin. Use brush #59 down the center of your nose (if you want to visually narrow it) and the top of the bow of the lips (to make them look fuller).

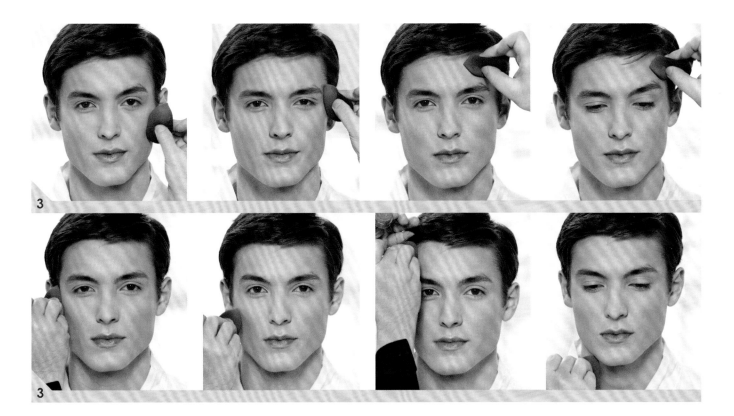

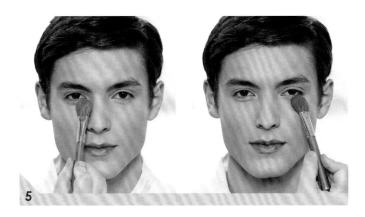

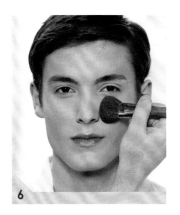

3. Apply your darkest, or contour, shade to the areas outside the oval, including all along your cheekbones, your temples, and along your jawline. By deepening the outside areas, you are visually helping those areas recede, making your face appear more narrow and oval.

4. Blend everything well.

5. Using brush #76 and a no-shimmer translucent highlight powder, set your highlight under your eyes and on top of your cheekbones, up the center of the nose, the center of the forehead, and the tip of the chin.

6. With powder brush #73, powder the rest of your face with a powder that matches your foundation exactly.

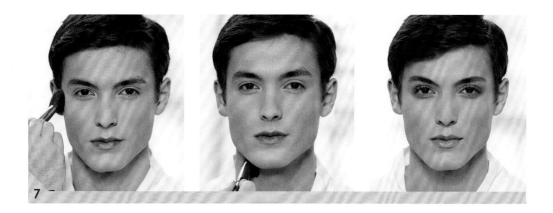

7.

7. With bronzing brush #73, reinforce your contour using a matte bronzer. Begin at the back of your cheekbone and sweep it forward to the apple of your cheek. Then, take the brush back toward your ear. This lays the color in place. Next, move your brush in the opposite direction (up and down) to blend well. Don't forget to add a little at the temples to help add shape and a glow. Sweep the bronzing powder up around the temples and eye socket. Finish by applying it along your jawline.

8. Using brush #11 and matte bronzing powder, sweep your brush up along the sides of your nose up into the beginning of your brow and crease. Apply across the tip of your nose, blending the edges well.

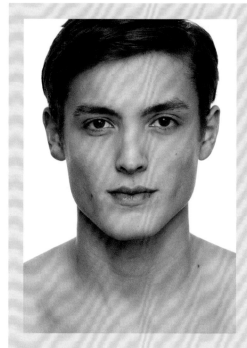

What a difference highlighting and contouring can make for his skin and face—and for yours.

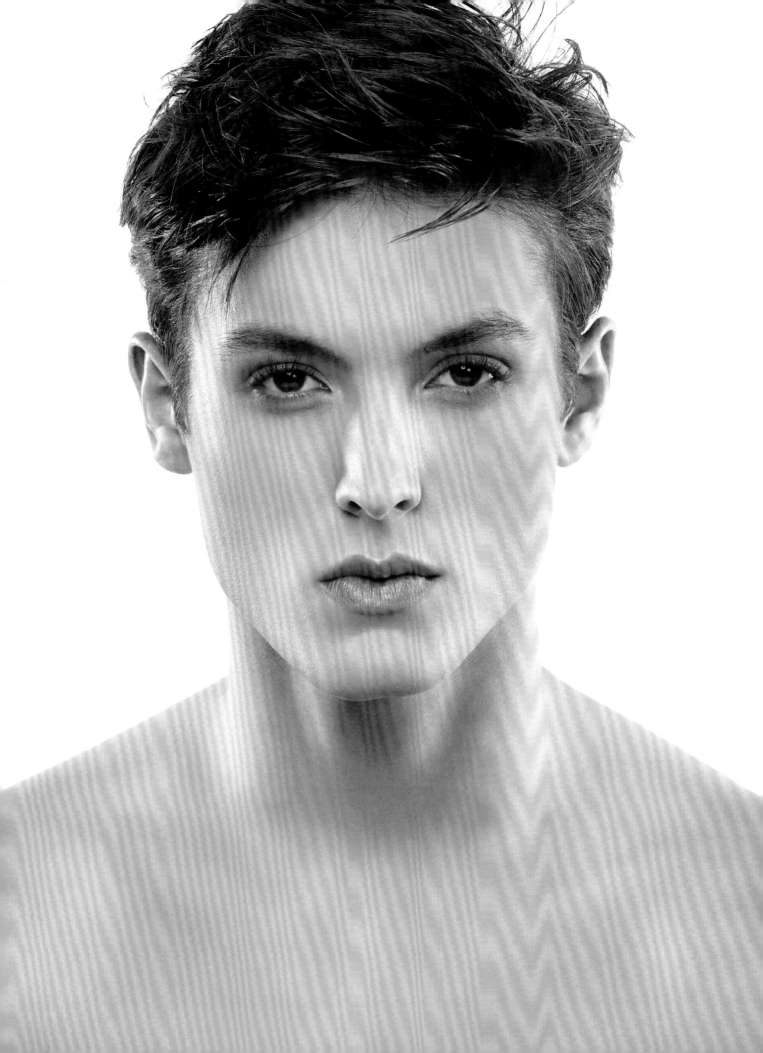

face shape

The way to sculpt your face depends on your face shape, but your goal is always the same: a more defined shape and beautiful glow. You do not need to know your face shape to make yourself look your best—you might even have a combination of face shapes. Simply envision the oval and then highlight the high points inside it and contour everything outside it. Everything about your face is unique, but no matter what, you can achieve a beautiful glow. Let's look at the best sculpting application for every face shape.

oval face

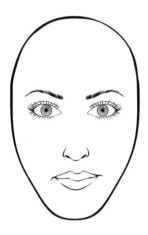

round face

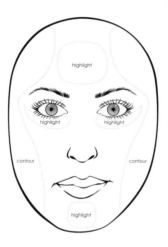

heart-shaped face

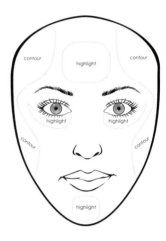

An oval face is considered the "perfect" face shape because of its symmetry. It is usually broader at the cheeks, tapering in slightly at both the forehead and chin. Because of its symmetry, you do not have to contour and highlight your face. If you pictured an oval around your face and nothing extended past it, your face is oval. That does not mean that you will not benefit from a generous dusting of bronzer along the cheekbones, temples, and even a bit on the tip of the chin. This will give you a glow and give your skin life. Feel free to experiment. An oval face can support most makeup trends, so have fun!

A round face is fuller and generally holds its youthful appearance longer than the other face shapes. It's shorter, wide, and has full cheeks and a rounded chin. When picturing your oval, some fullness will extend out past the oval. Contouring that fullness away will narrow the appearance of your face.

If you have a round face:

- Highlight your forehead, underneath your eyes, on top of your cheekbones, and the center of your chin to draw attention to the center of your face.

- Contour your temples, cheeks, and jawline with a foundation and/or bronzer that is darker than your skin tone to create the illusion of an oval.

The heart-shaped face looks like an inverted triangle: it's wider at the forehead and cheeks, curving down to a narrow chin. When you picture your oval, notice a fullness extending at your temples and cheeks, and contour and soften the fullness in these areas. This is the least common face shape.

If you have a heart-shaped face:

- Highlight your chin to help broaden it. Highlight your forehead and underneath your eyes, just on top of the cheekbones, to draw attention to the center of your face.

- Contour your temples and cheeks to diminish the width of this portion of your face.

square face

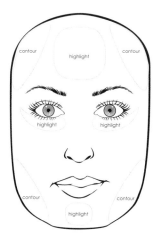

pear-shaped face

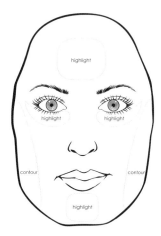

long face

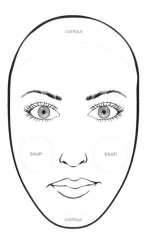

I consider this shape to be one of the most beautiful and the most photogenic because it suggests strength and the features are usually symmetrically balanced. A square-shaped face is the same width at the forehead, the cheeks, and the jaw. When envisioning your oval around this face shape, you will be left with four corners to contour or soften.

If you have a square face:

- Highlight the center of your forehead, underneath your eyes, on top of your cheekbones, and the tip of your chin to draw attention to the middle of your face.

- Contour your hairline at the two corners by your temples and the two corners of your jaw.

- Apply blush on the apples of your cheeks to help draw attention away from the corners of the square and widen the area to make it appear more oval.

The pear-shaped face is narrow at the temples and forehead and wider at the cheeks and jawline. When envisioning your oval, the area at your cheeks and jaw will extend out past your oval, and that is the area you need to minimize. This is the most common face shape.

If you have a pear-shaped face:

- Highlight your forehead to create the illusion of width and highlight underneath your eyes, on top of your cheekbones, and the tip of your chin.

- Contour from your cheeks down along your jaw to minimize the width of this area.

The long face has high cheekbones, a high and deep forehead, and a strong, chiseled jawline.

If you have a long face:

- Never highlight the oval area of your face! This will make your face appear even longer.

- Brush a bit of bronzer across your chin and across your forehead at your hairline to help make your face look shorter.

- Be generous with your blush and place a lot of color on the apples of your cheeks. This will help widen and shorten your face. When applying your blush, start closer in on the apples of the cheeks and brush outward across your face.

- Bangs can help shorten the length of your face.

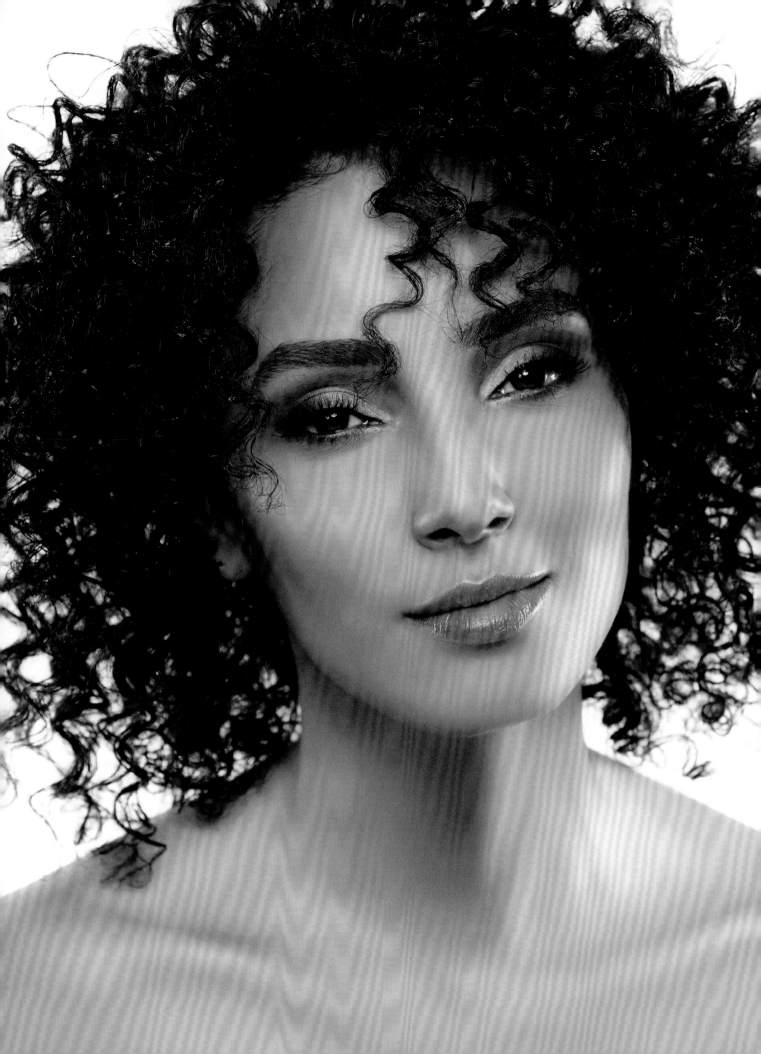

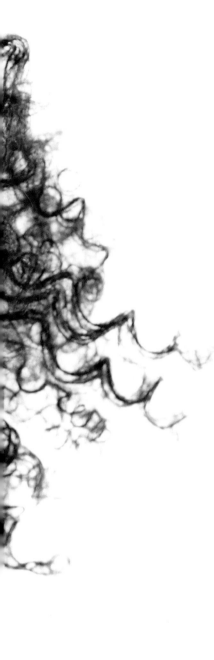

chapter 5

eye basics

Your eyebrows, the frame to your face, give you your expression. They can make you look harsh or soften you. Don't underestimate their importance.

Fuller brows make you look younger, and they tend to fit more face shapes. So, one of my best bits of advice is, don't go wild and rip them all out. You will want them later in life, and if you tweeze them out over a long time, they may not grow back.

And don't follow eyebrow fashion trends; they come and go, and they're not always right for your face shape. Don't try to make your brows look like someone else's! Your brow shape is individual to you, so embrace it. For instance, if your brows grow very straight, you will never have a high arch. Some people have a natural arch; some don't. Whatever your natural shape, there is a way to groom your brows to make them look amazing.

Before we begin, gather your tools: a good pair of tweezers, a brow brush, and a small pair of scissors.

trim your eyebrows

Let's begin by evaluating your brows.

First, are they too dense or heavy? Trimming can soften them if they are. It will completely change the way your eyebrow hairs lie on your face.

Often, brow hairs are longer than they appear because the tips of the hairs are lighter in color, and when they reach a certain length, they tend to curl. By trimming them, you trim away some of the density and that slight curl, so they lie down more neatly.

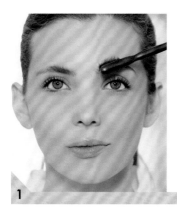
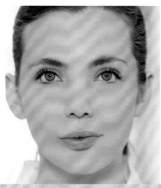
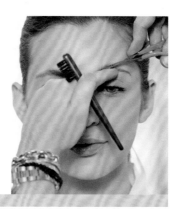

1. To trim your brow: Brush your eyebrows up and snip any stray hairs that extend past the upper brow line.

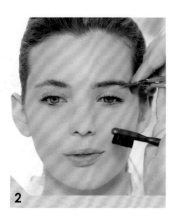

2. Brush them down and snip any unruly hairs that extend past the lower brow line.

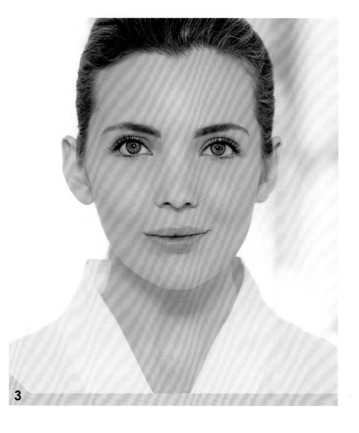

3. Now brush them back into place. Notice how much better they lie and how much softer they look on your face.

If you need to trim your brows, do it before you start to tweeze. Otherwise, you might ruin your brow line by tweezing away hairs that should have stayed but were simply too long.

tweeze your eyebrows

The best time to tweeze your brows is after a steamy shower, when it's a lot less painful because your pores are already open. Try to tweeze in natural light; you'll be able to see what you're doing much better. Always tweeze in the direction your hair grows. If you don't, it can damage the hair follicle, and the hair might not grow back properly—sticking straight out rather than lying down, for example.

If you have naturally full brows, you never want to tweeze them pencil-thin because your face needs a fuller brow. Shape them and groom them, just don't over-tweeze them.

Tweezing your brows to look like each other can be very difficult. Very few people have brows that grow exactly symmetrically. If you fully tweeze one eyebrow first, you may never make the other match it no matter how much you work, simply because of the way it grows. If you do what I call "tweezing from side to side" instead, it will help you make them more even. Start by tweezing a couple of hairs out of one brow, then switch to the other, tweeze a couple out of it, and switch back to the first. This way you can constantly reevaluate what needs to be tweezed, and the frequent comparison will help you get them more even.

How do you determine where to start?

By locating three key points of reference, we will know where and what to tweeze.

I have been trying to grow my brows back in to look fuller, but it seems that no matter what I do, they are not getting any thicker. What can—or should— I do?

If you are trying to grow your brows back in fuller, you must leave them alone and tweeze nothing for at least two to six months. Otherwise, you will tweeze a hair out that you think shouldn't be there, but will need to be when your brows fill in. Also, take heart: even if you have over-tweezed for years, there are now products available that will help promote new hair growth, so you can even grow back hairs that you thought were gone for good.

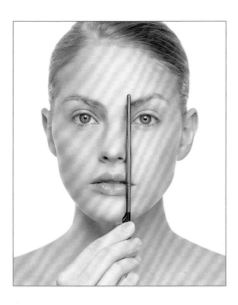

Point A. Hold a pencil or the handle of a brush vertically against the side of your nose, noting where it meets the brow. That is where your eyebrow should begin. Keep in mind the width you put between your brows will affect how wide the bridge of your nose appears. The wider the space between your brows, the wider your nose can look; the narrower the space, the narrower your nose will look.

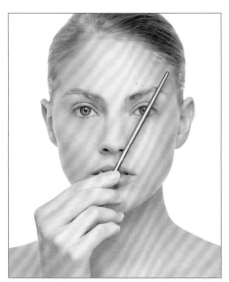

Point B. Hold the handle against your nostril and move it diagonally across the outer half of the iris of your eye. Note where the handle meets your brow: This is the best place for the peak of your arch. If you tweeze from point A to point B, tapering the line slightly toward the peak, you will create the ideal shape for your brow. It is a gentle taper, using the natural width at the beginning of your brow (point A) and slowly tapering it as you get to the arch (point B).

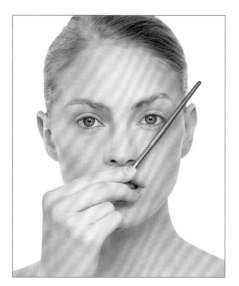

Point C. Place the handle against your nostril again, but this time, extend it diagonally to the outer corner of your eye. Where it meets the brow is the best place for your brow to end. If you tweeze from point B to point C, tapering the line even thinner, you will create the best brow shape for your face. Once again, it is a slow taper from point B to point C, not a drastic change.

tip: *Make sure you tweeze one hair at a time. Tweezing clusters could cause bald spots.*

what to color your brow

Did you know that you can choose a brow color as easily as a hair color? The basic rule of thumb is that it should pretty closely match your hair color (whether natural or chosen). Let's elaborate a little bit, though, because it's not just as simple as that. Here are the perfect brow colors for each hair color:

- **light blonde:** the same shade as your hair or one shade darker

- **medium to dark blonde:** the same color as your hair

- **auburn:** the same color as your hair

- **light brown:** the same color as your hair or one shade lighter

- **medium to dark brown:** the same color as your hair or one shade lighter

- **very dark brown to black:** one shade lighter than your hair color, to soften the look of your brows and prevent them from making you look too harsh

- **silver or gray:** a blonde or soft taupe for ivory or beige skin tones or a light golden brown for bronze or ebony skin tones. A silver or gray brow color to match your hair would just wash you out and make you look older. Another option is to have them dyed; they make special products to do this.

Just a reminder: Brow color products are specifically designed for their job. Eyebrow pencils are duller in color, usually with no sheen, and have a somewhat waxier texture than eyeliner pencils do. Eyebrow powder is duller and more matte than eye shadow. Make sure you are using products designed to do the job at hand.

tip: *When you have your hair colored, ask your colorist to tint your brows to match. This will ensure that your brows match your hair.*

how to apply brow color

The goal when applying brow color is to mimic your natural brows. You want to draw short feather-like hair strokes, meant to imitate natural eyebrow hairs, as you apply the color, never a straight solid line. Here are the best application techniques for each type of brow color and grooming product you might choose (see page 19).

eyebrow pencil

An eyebrow pencil is probably the most commonly used and certainly the most portable coloring tool. The sharper the point, the better the application, so sharpen your pencil before you start.

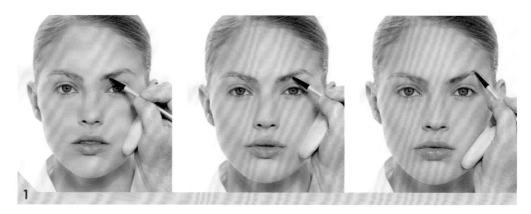

1. With your pencil, make short, feathery, hair-like strokes, angled in the same direction as the hairs' growth. Your strokes should mimic natural brow hairs (never draw a solid straight line).

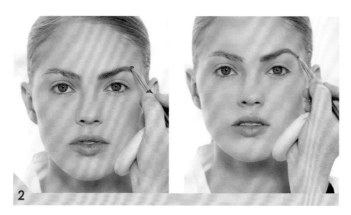

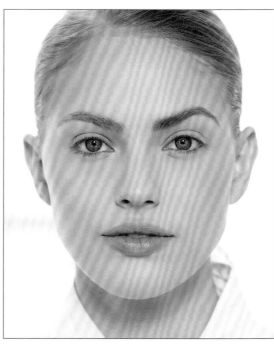

2. Using a small stiff-angled brush, go over the pencil strokes you just made, using the same short strokes. This will blend the color even more, making it look natural.

powder

Powder is probably the easiest of all brow color options to apply, and it also looks the most natural. It is perfect if your brows don't need much filling in, but you want to define and refine them. It is also the quickest and easiest to apply because there is only one step—you apply and blend at the same time. Dip your short, stiff-angled brush in product and draw short, feathery, hair-like strokes angled in the same direction as the hairs' growth. Remember: no straight lines, just short, feathery strokes.

crème/pomade

This will give you the most coverage, but it is the hardest to master, so give it some practice. It's a great choice for you if you need a lot of coverage due to over-plucking or chemotherapy, or if you just really want dramatic brows. (However, I prefer the powder-on-pencil technique on the next page.)

1. Using a short, stiff-angled brush, apply your crème/pomade using short, feathery, hair-like strokes.

2. Make sure to always follow your crème with powder brow color, using the exact same application method. The powder will set the crème and help it last all day. Most of your pomade formulas won't necessarily have to be followed by a powder because they dry to a finish that the crèmes do not.

tip: *Sharpen your eyebrow pencil each time you use it. The sharper the point, the better the application.*

pencil and powder for more coverage

If you have scars in your eyebrows or brows that just are not there, you will need more coverage. You could use a crème, but I prefer to layer eyebrow pencil and eyebrow powder together because it looks most natural. I almost always layer pencil and powder when apply brow color. It helps your brows last longer and look more natural.

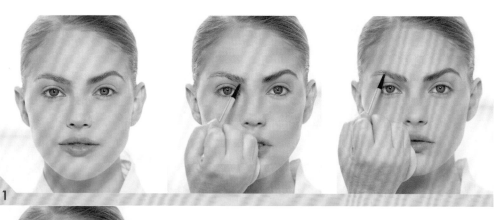

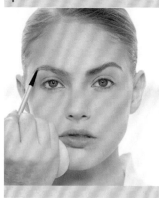

1. With your pencil, make short, feathery, hair-like strokes angled in the same direction as the hairs' growth. Your strokes are meant to mimic natural brow hairs (never draw a solid straight line). I usually use a pencil that is lighter than the natural brow color to make it look softer and more natural.

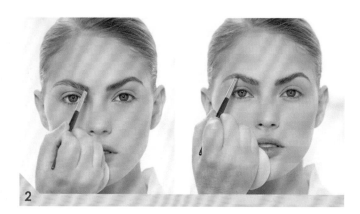

2. With a small stiff-angled brush, go over the pencil you just applied using the same short strokes. This will blend your color even more, making it look extremely natural.

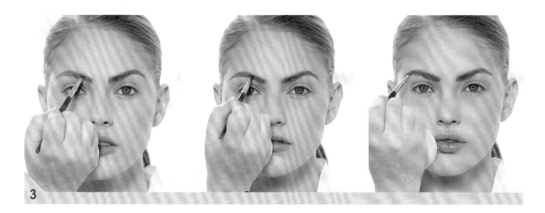

3. Dip your brush in eyebrow powder and apply it once again using short, feathery, hair-like strokes angled in the same direction as the hairs' growth. I usually choose a powder that's the exact brow color so it gives a subtler effect when layered with the lighter pencil. Make sure you cover the entire brow. The powder and pencil layered together will give you more complete coverage, help the color last longer, and look more natural.

Whichever method you prefer, always finish by using a brow brush (my favorite is shaped like a toothbrush) to brush all your brow hairs upward and outward. This will ensure that your brow hairs are lying in place, and it will blend your color beautifully to give you an absolutely natural effect. If you have wild, unruly brows and need help keeping them tamed during the day, you can end with a brow gel. It acts like hairspray for the brows.

I have a lot of brow hairs, but they are so light that you can't see them. My eyebrow pencil always looks unnatural because my natural blonde brow hairs lie over the pencil, causing it to look fake. What can I do so that my brows are defined yet appear natural?

The answer for you is tinting your brows. Have a professional at a salon tint (darken) them so they will show. They make products to specifically use in the eye area. I will say, though, this color tends to fade quickly, so have them tinted a shade darker than you think you might want so that the color will last longer. After your brows are tinted, you will need less eyebrow pencil, and what you do use will look completely natural.

apply your eye shadow

I almost always make the eyes the focus of the face. It is often said that they are the windows to the soul. What are yours saying about you? Applying color correctly to your eyes can go a long way toward making your signature statement to the world. With eye makeup, it should always be your goal to bring out your eyes and help them grab everyone's attention. When someone looks at you, you want that person to think you look beautiful today, not that your eye makeup does.

Let's start with how to apply eye makeup on a basic eye. It's not the perfect application for every eye shape, but it is a place to start when you are first learning to apply makeup.

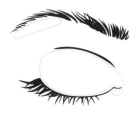 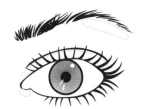

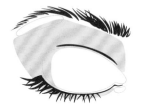 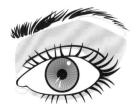

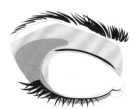 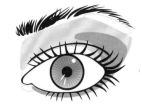

You have a basic eye if your eyes are one eye width apart—that is, the space between your eyes is the same width as one of your eyes. Also, when you look in the mirror, you'll see the entire eyelid, from lash line to crease. You'll have a defined crease all the way across, and you'll have a clear and definite amount of space above the crease with a normal, not overly prominent, brow bone. Let's talk about how to make a basic shaped eye look it's best.

The diagram at left shows where to place your highlight, midtone, and contour shades.

application: basic eye

Your first goal when applying eye shadow is to give the eyelid shape by visually pushing away the areas you don't want to see and bringing forward the areas you do. That will also help you achieve your second goal, which is to define and open up your eyes. Proper eye makeup application will make your eyes appear more open, so you look awake.

It takes three shades to shape the eye: a highlight, a midtone, and a contour shade. The basic rule is that everything you highlight will become more visible, and everything you contour or darken will recede. Using three shades creates a subtle visual trick to help bring out one of your most beautiful features and help draw attention to your eyes rather than your eyelids. Let's learn more about these three shades.

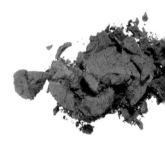

Your highlight shade is the lightest of the three eye shadows. Everything you highlight comes forward visually. How dramatically it comes forward depends on the shade and finish you select. A matte finish will give you a much subtler look than a shimmer finish. I usually use a shimmer highlight on deep-set eyes because it opens up the eye more than a matte shade. Also, the lighter the highlight shade is, the more dramatic your result will be. A softer or more flesh-toned shade will give you a less dramatic look.

Your midtone shade is the most important shade. It is the middle shade of your three eye shadow colors, deeper than your highlight shade and lighter than your contour shade. It's the first step in the blending process and in creating definition in the crease of the eye. This shade should be the most natural—an extension of your skin. You'll change your highlight and contour colors more often than your midtone shade. Most of the time, it is best for your midtone color to have a matte finish, but it doesn't always have to. A matte finish gives it a more subtle and natural appearance. The application of your midtone will start the reshaping of your eyelids because everything we add depth to will visually recede away from us.

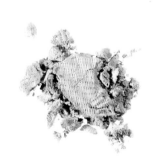

The contour shade is the deepest of the three shades. It's not necessarily stark or dark—it can even be metallic—but it is the deepest color. The contour eye shadow is the shade you can have fun with and change with your mood. You'll find that most makeup lines offer plenty of contour colors because they are the most eye catching and exciting to use. Your contour shade does the most dramatic reshaping of your eyelid because of its depth. This shade really helps define the eyes.

Now that we have a better understanding of our three shades, here's where to put them on the eyelid:

1. Apply the highlight shade to your eyelid and if you want to, your brow bone (the area immediately underneath your brow's arch). However, don't apply it all the way from the lash line to the brow because that can be detrimental to most eye shapes.

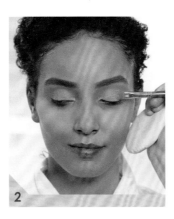

2. For more pop, start with shimmery beige crème-to-powder eye shadow because layering a crème and a powder will make your highlight more dramatic. Using your #22 highlight brush, apply your crème shadow to your lid only.

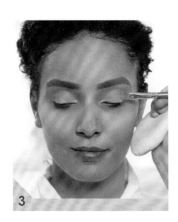

3. With the same brush, layer on a shimmery gold and a matte flesh over the crème. The reason for layering the two is you will still get the shine from the shimmer while making it opaque by adding the matte, giving you even more coverage. Just keep in mind when loading the brush that the color you touch first will be on top, so touch the shimmer shadow first and then the matte; that way the matte will be against your skin.

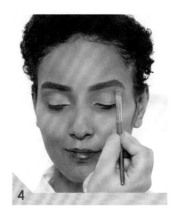

4. With your #22 highlight brush, apply the matte flesh eye shadow to your brow bone.

5. Curl your eyelashes and do your first layer of mascara now (see page 136). This will give it time to dry so you can apply more layers without them clumping, and your highlight shade won't drip down on your eyelashes and wash out your mascara.

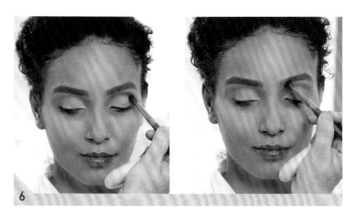

6. With your #11 midtone brush, apply a matte ginger midtone eye shadow, starting from the outside corner of the eyelid, so that area will get the most midtone color because the first place you lay your brush receives the highest concentration of color. Gently move your brush along the crease into the inside corner of your eyelid (from the outside corner all the way across to the inside corner). For a very defined crease, you can apply a few more layers of your midtone shade (feel free to layer for more definition).

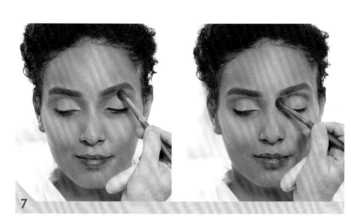

7. With your #16 blending brush, blend your midtone so that there are no hard edges. To create a perfectly blended eye, you need a clean brush that is only used for blending. You cannot blend with the brush you apply color with; it will only create mud.

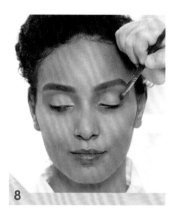

8. Using your #30 contour brush, apply more of your midtone to the outer corner of your eyelid to close it in.

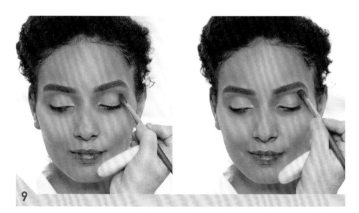

9. With your #16 blending brush, blend out the shadow that you just applied, blending up toward your crease and in toward the center of your eyelid. Keep the blend tight so you don't darken the lid too much.

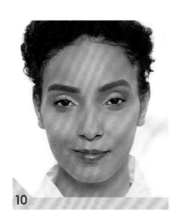

10. You can see, comparing one eye with midtone and one without, how much shaping just your midtone does. It does 85 percent of the heavy lifting. I could just line this eye and apply more layers of mascara and it would look finished—not dramatic, but finished.

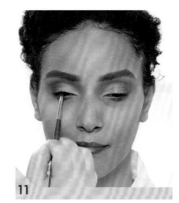

11. I like to create the illusion of thicker eyelashes and start the lash line definition by applying a matte black shadow at the base of the lash line, in between the eyelashes. Using your #41 detail eye liner brush, push matte black shadow into your upper lash line starting from you outside corner and working your way all the way across to the inner corner.

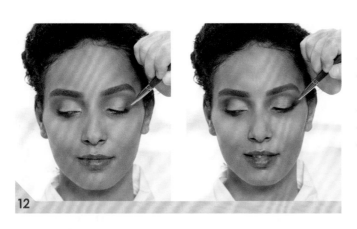

12. This step is optional, but it can help create more depth at the lash line, which will help you create a dark-to-light gradation of color. Layering a crème and powder shadow will make it grab darker, so using another #22 highlight brush, apply a dark copper crème eye shadow all along your lash line in the outer corner of your lid.

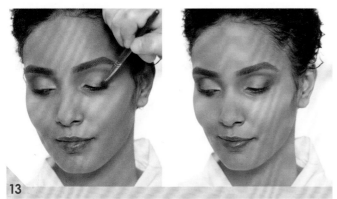

13. With your #30 contour brush, layer a dark matte brown in the outer corner of the eyelid at the base of the lash line, on top of the crème.

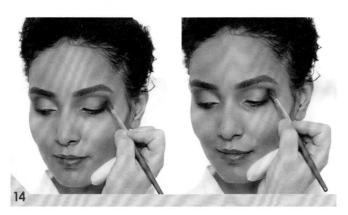

14. With your #16 blending brush, blend the color up toward the crease and in toward the inner part of the lid.

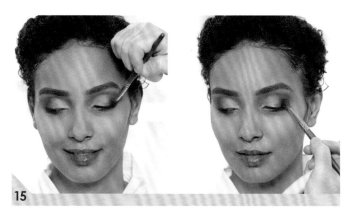

15. Keep layering on color with your #30 contour brush and blending it out with your #16 blending brush until you reach your desired intensity. Your goal is to blend the color up into the outer portion of the crease and blend it inward (about a third or, at most, halfway across). You want to create a gradation of color, with the outer corner of the eye being the darkest and becoming lighter as you move in toward the inside of the eyelid. By layering your contour shade on top of your midtone shade, you'll get the blended, defined look you want.

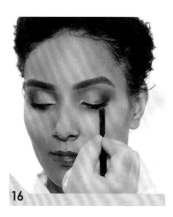

16. Create your final upper lash line definition: Using black eyeliner, line your upper lash line (see page 130).

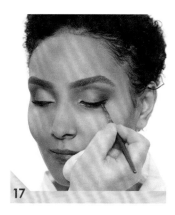

17. Using your #42 eye liner brush, smooth out your liner.

18. For more definition, apply another layer of mascara now, so the layer has time to dry. Optional: This is the time to apply false eyelashes (see page 188).

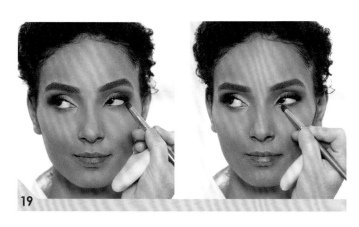

19. With your #13 detail eye shadow brush, apply your midtone all along your lower lash line. Once again, start your application from the outside corner, sweeping it across to the inside corner. Applying midtone here before you apply eyeliner or your contour shade will help create a blend because you are building depth of color creating a gradation. This way you won't have stark dark liner against pale or light skin.

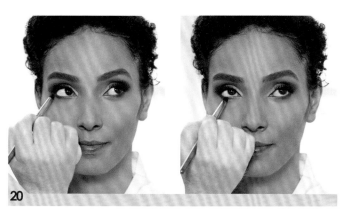

20. With the same brush, apply your contour color underneath and along the lower lash line to define your eyes. Blending it over your eye pencil will also help give you a softer, subtler lined effect. If I were going to use pencil along the lower lash line, I would apply it after the midtone and before the contour. For this look, I only used midtone and contour along the lower lash line to create definition.

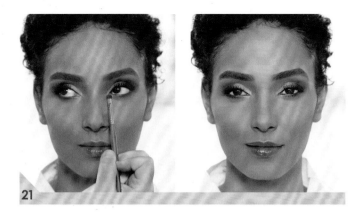

21. With your #14 eye shadow brush, apply your highlight shade to the inside corner of the lower lash line. This will really help open up your eyes, making them appear larger.

22. Finish by applying the third and final layer of mascara to your top lashes (or by blending into your false eyelashes with mascara) and a layer to your bottom lashes.

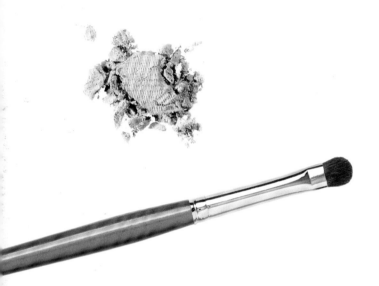

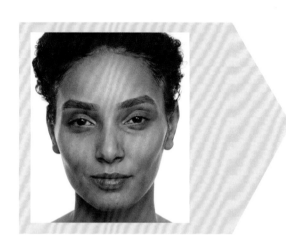

How can I get my eye shadow to blend better, go on more smoothly, and last longer?

I always apply concealer and powder to the eyelids before applying eye shadow. It will get rid of any discoloration on your eyelid and give you a clean canvas on which to artfully paint your eye shadow. It will also help all the shades you use look clearer and truer in tone. This technique also helps your eye shadows blend more easily and wear longer. I know some people think foundation will work for this, but there are some formulas that could cause your eye shadow to crease (because they contain moisture), and foundation will not cover discoloration and create a clean canvas the way a concealer will. There are also products out there called eye primers that will create a perfect surface for you to apply color to—they help prevent creasing and prevent the natural oils in your eyelids from reacting with the eye shadows, causing them to build up in the crease. If you use an eye primer, you should still follow it with concealer and powder because the primer will not cover all discoloration, and eye primer can hinder the all-important blend-ability of your eye shadows.

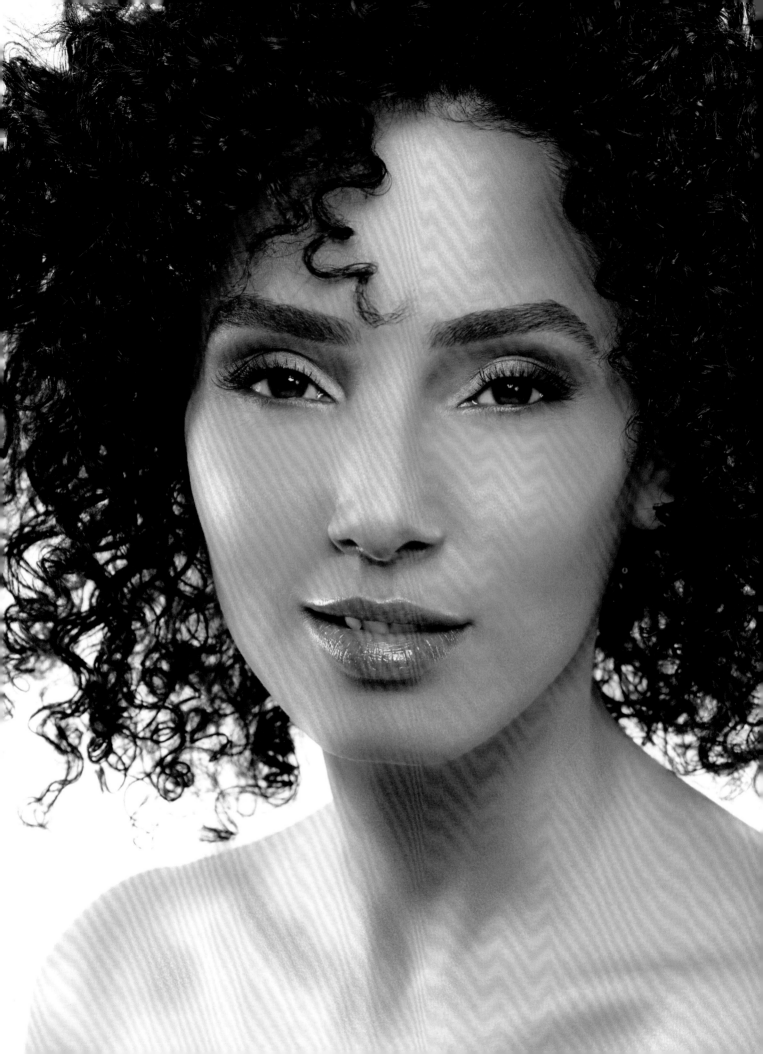

apply your eyeliner

Eyeliner can go a long way toward defining your eyes—opening them up and drawing attention to them—but if used incorrectly, it will close them down and make them look smaller. There are several ways to define your eyes when lining them, but first let's set some ground rules:

- If you line along your bottom lash line, you must line across your top lash line. If you don't, the depth along the bottom will pull the eye down without the balance along the top, and your eyes will look older and tired.

- You can line along the top lash line without lining along the bottom. I usually like a little definition along the bottom, even if it is just a little of your eye shadow contour color, but you don't need it.

- You can skip eyeliner if you want a soft, natural look. You can also get a natural look by taking an eyeliner brush and a dark eye shadow and just adding a little soft definition at your lash line. Using an eye shadow instead of eyeliner is much subtler. It will give you a little definition without making your eyes looked lined.

- The color along your bottom lash line should never be deeper in depth than along your top lash line, or once again it will just drag your eye down. I find that a lot of people want more definition along their top lash line than they do along the bottom, and this is always okay. For example, you could use deep brown eyeliner along your top lash line while choosing a soft bronze for along the bottom; it just makes it look softer and subtler.

For any lining option, your goal is: to create definition and make your eyes the focus of your look. As you age, you still want to define your eyes; it will wake your face up and create a wide-eyed, youthful expression. I am constantly asked where to apply color. How far in do you go with color? Where do you start and where do you stop? Where should you line? How thick a line should you create?

A simple rule of thumb works for all eye shapes (as shown in the images opposite, at top). Along your top lash line, you want your definition to start at the inside corner of your eye, where you want the liner to be thinnest. It should gradually become wider as you apply it across to the outer corner of the eye. This will create definition without closing in the eye. Along your lower lash line, you want the color to be most intense in the outer corner, fading as you move toward the inside corner. Bring it all the way across the bottom lash line, but make sure it fades in intensity from the outer corner to the inner corner. Drawing the same thickness all the way across the top lash line can close in your eyes and make them appear smaller. You want a gradation of color along the bottom lash line for definition and attention. Your color should be as close to the lash line as possible. Don't let any skin show between your eyelashes and your eyeliner!

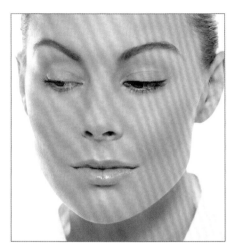 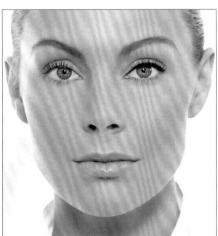 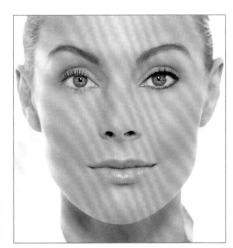

Now let's talk about application options. Most often, I choose to line or create my definition around the eye with nothing more than the correct brush and a dark eye shadow. Not only is it the easiest to apply, it also creates the subtlest effect.

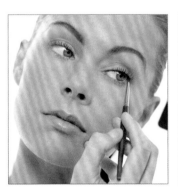 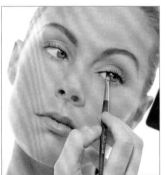 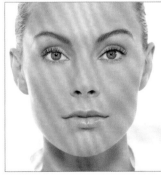

tip: *The professional secret to creating definition along the lash line is to get the color right into the base of the eyelashes (especially along the top lash line). There is a little secret trick many of us makeup pros do that can create definition like no other: You simply take black eye shadow and carefully push it into the base of your eyelashes using a fine-tipped brush. This defines the eyes and makes your eyelashes look thicker without making your eyes appear lined. You could take a pencil and scrub it into the base of your eyelashes as well, but I find it easier to use eye shadow and a brush.*

powder

1. Dip a dry eyeliner brush (see page 37) in your powder eye shadow and tap the excess off.

2. Place the brush along your top lash line and sweep it from the outside corner in toward the inside corner. This will give you a subtle wash of color along the lash line.

3. Dip the brush in your eye shadow again and tap off the excess.

4. Starting from the outside corner (because the first place we lay the brush will get the highest concentration of color), sweep the color along your lower lash line, all the way across. This will automatically create a fading of color from the outer corner (the deepest) to the inner corner (the lightest).

pencil

The application of eyeliner pencil can be difficult. Here are some tricks to make it easier:

1. Don't feel like you have to apply your eyeliner in one straight, solid line. Begin at the outside corner of your eye and draw small, feather-like strokes or dashes, connecting each one as you move toward the inside of the eye.

2. You can make eyeliner pencil look even better by using an eyeliner brush to blend across the line you just created, making it look like one solid, mistake-free line. I also suggest this professional technique: Before you use your brush to blend, dip it in a little eye shadow. This will help the line look more smudged and soften its appearance. You could use a shade of eye shadow that matches your eyeliner, or you could choose a different shade to customize your liner color.

3. With your eyeliner pencil, starting at the outside corner of your lower lash line, begin to draw small, feather-like strokes, connecting each one as you move toward the inside corner of the eye. It will look more natural if you draw into the actual base of your eyelashes rather than just below them.

4. Blend the line with your brush. I find it especially effective to use an eye shadow when blending. The main benefit is that the outside corner—the first place you lay the brush—gets the highest concentration of color, and as you sweep your brush across, it blends the liner, helping it fade as you move inward. When you are finished, it will be darkest at the outside corner and fade toward the inside corner, which is your goal.

liquid, crème, and gel

These three types of eyeliner are similar in their appearance and application. They will give you the most dramatic effect—think Audrey Hepburn and her signature cat-eyed eyeliner look! One advantage of liquid, crème, and gel eyeliners is that they usually have great staying power.

You can only use these eyeliners along the top lash line. Never use them along the bottom lash line—they will look too harsh and stark. If you want color along your lower lash line when using liquid, crème, or gel eyeliner along your top lash line, use pencil or powder for your lower lash definition. With these three formulas, practice makes perfect: The more you use them, the better you will get at applying them.

How to apply them: With your applicator (if you're using a liquid, it comes with a brush or felt tip; with crème or gel, you will need an eyeliner brush), starting at the inside corner of your top lash line, slowly move across the lash line. Make sure your line is its most narrow at the inside corner, gradually getting thicker as you reach the outside corner. As your brush reaches the outside corner, you can give it a little kick upward.

cake

This is a powder that looks much like an eye shadow in its container. It is much heavier and more highly pigmented than an eye shadow, though. Cake eyeliner is easy to apply and gives you a similar effect to a liquid, crème, or gel. You apply it the same way as the other three, only you need to dampen your brush before beginning. Just make sure you have the right brush for the job (see page 37).

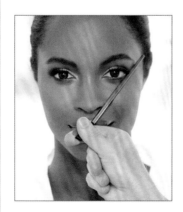

curl your eyelashes

I have five words to say about eyelashes: curl, curl, curl, curl, and curl. There is no quicker, cheaper, faster facelift than curling your eyelashes. It opens your eyes, lifts your lids, and makes your eyes look bigger. If you don't think you need to curl, just look at the before-and-after pictures below. All she has done is curl her eyelashes. You can see how much it has lifted her eye and made it appear more open.

Nowadays you have many curling options, from the classic crimp curler to a detailed precision eyelash curler to one of my favorites, the heated eyelash curler. No matter what your choice is, just remember to curl!

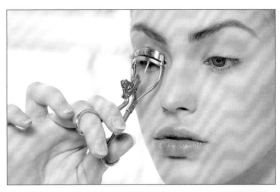

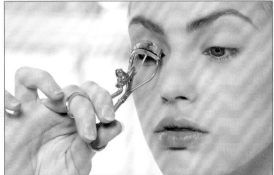

If your choice is a classic crimp curler, it is fast and easy, but make sure the tool you use is fairly new. If you use an eyelash curler for more than a year, it can get out of alignment and cut your eyelashes. Throw out the one from high school; it's time to by a new one! You need to replace a crimp curler every year and change the rubber piece every six months. The trick to using a crimp curler is to crimp your eyelashes more than just once at the lash line. Instead, "walk" the eyelash curler up the length of your eyelashes, taking care to close, open, and move the eyelash curler up several times until you reach the end. Some women can crimp once, some three times; the point is to walk it out and crimp it as many times as you can until you reach the end. This method creates a curve rather than a crimp and will help your eye-lashes stay curled.

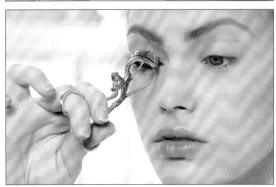

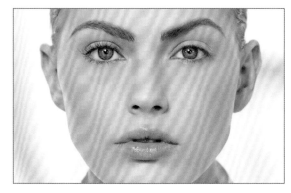

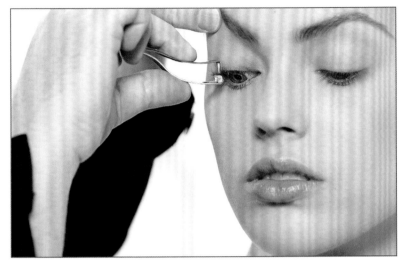

A detailed precision eyelash curler works the same way a classic crimp curler works; you crimp it down on the lash and it curls. The big difference is the size: It is only about a fourth the width of the classic version, making it easier to get right at the base of the eyelashes. Start at the base of the eyelashes and crimp as you walk it out to the ends, just as you did with the classic crimp curler.

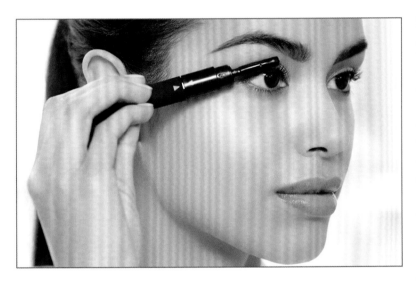

If you're afraid of crimp-style eyelash curlers, you're in luck: There is now an alternative eyelash-curling tool, a heated eyelash curler. This tool is used after you've applied mascara. It uses your mascara as a curling catalyst—an excellent feature because applying mascara can slightly uncurl your eyelashes. Starting at the base of your eyelashes, work it back and forth from side to side, so your eyelashes can fall into the grooves of the curler. Now push up and twist the curler in toward your lid, and your eyelashes will be curled to perfection—no crimping needed!

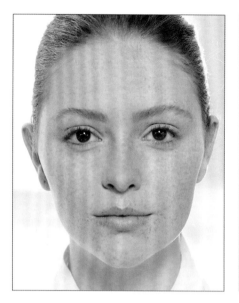 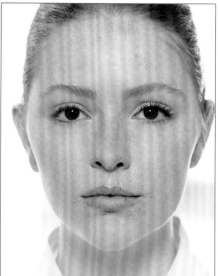

Curl your eyelashes, as shown above left. Then add a layer of mascara. Even a single layer of mascara, shown right, can make an enormous difference in starting to define your eyes. It helps open them up and gives you the attention you are looking for.

layer on your mascara

Curled, thick, dark, luscious eyelashes equal young and beautiful. Mascara is everyone's favorite way to add definition to the eyes. I recommend applying several coats to define and open your eyes because layering it will give you the most dramatic definition. If you have allergies or are concerned about getting teary-eyed, you can make any application waterproof by making your final coat a layer of waterproof mascara.

Here's the best way to apply several coats of mascara to build eyelashes that last:

1. Curl your eyelashes with a crimp-style eyelash curler, opening up the eyes and making them appear larger. (If you opt to use a heated curler, do so once you've applied your mascara and it's thoroughly dried.)

2. Pull the mascara wand out of the tube and wipe the brush against the opening or on a paper towel to remove any excess product. Don't be afraid of cleaning too much product off—there is plenty on there!

3. Apply the small amount that is left on the brush to your eyelashes.

4. Using an eyelash comb, comb your eyelashes before the mascara dries. This will help keep your eyelashes well separated and prevent them from clumping.

5. Let each coat of mascara dry between applications. This could take a couple of minutes, so be patient, but each coat must be completely dry. If you do not wait for each layer to dry, your eyelashes will clump. This is also why I like to apply my first layer when it has plenty of time to dry before the second layer.

6. After one coat is dry, pull out your wand, clean it off, and apply the next coat. Repeat as necessary.

The trick to mastering multiple-coat application is making sure to apply very thin coats, letting each dry completely between coats. I almost always apply three coats to the top lash line and one coat to the bottom.

tip: *No matter what the formula, when you pull a mascara wand out of its tube, it will likely have more product on it than you want (especially if you're layering). It is always best to clean the excess off your brush before you apply mascara.*

There is no rule saying you must apply mascara to your bottom lashes; it is a matter of personal preference. When I first started my makeup career many, many years ago, I never used mascara on the bottom lashes (it was not in fashion), but now I almost always do (for the eye definition). The one time I might try to convince you not to use mascara along your lower lash line would be if your eyelashes are very sparse because defining them will only accentuate how sparse they are.

Here's a trick of the trade: If you don't use mascara on your eyelashes, make sure you smudge your eyeliner well because that is what mascara would do: break up the line, making it look much more natural.

Then there is the ever-present question: black versus brown versus a color (such as blue, purple, etc.). This is something I feel very strongly about because your eyelashes are so important for giving your eyes definition. For me it is always black. If I'm going to have a party, I'm going to have a big party! Black will give you the most definition. I'm not opposed to brown or black/brown, especially if they make you feel more comfortable. Choose one of them if you want a softer result (less definition). Colored mascara is always a no for me; it does not look natural, and it does nothing for your eyes.

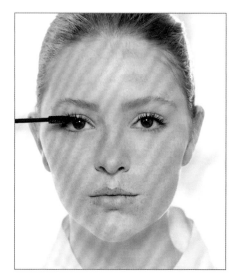

For thicker eyelashes: Start at the base of the eyelashes and hold your mascara wand in a horizontal position, moving it from side to side as you work your way up to the end. This technique makes the mascara particles attach to the sides of your eyelashes, making them appear thicker.

tip: *Coat your eyelashes with mascara at the inside corners and the very outer corners. These are the two areas that many women miss.*

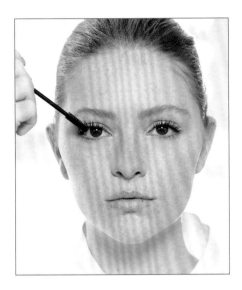

For longer eyelashes: Hold your mascara wand in a vertical position. Starting at the base of the lash line, pull the wand up and out to the end. The particles will attach to the ends of your eyelashes, making them appear longer.

If you want both—and you deserve both!—simply apply multiple layers each way. For example, apply your first coat thick (horizontally) and then let it dry. Apply your next coat (vertically) so it lengthens, let it dry, and so on. If you want to waterproof your eyelashes, just make your final layer waterproof.

tip: *Two or three thinly applied coats of mascara are far more effective than a single clumpy one.*

My mascara always seems to smear and smudge, even if I wear a waterproof variety. What can I do to keep my mascara from smudging and smearing?

If you are having problems with mascara smudging and smearing even with a waterproof formula, chances are good that the mascara is not adhering to your eyelashes. There are a couple of things to try: First, powder (with loose or pressed powder) under your eyes to set your foundation and concealer. Not setting the two can cause your mascara to smear. Secondly, make sure the mascara can grab onto your eyelashes. Be careful when applying your moisturizer and eye crèmes not to get them on your eyelashes (it's very easy to do accidentally). If you do, the mascara won't be able to adhere, and it will smudge and smear.

Q & A

how to conquer every eye shape

Now that you know how to apply makeup to a basic eye, let's explore other eye shapes. Most eyes are a combination of shapes, but usually one shape stands out. You still need the same three ingredients—your highlight, midtone, and contour. The general area of placement is the same; we just shift it slightly to push back what we don't want to see and bring forward what we do. Each eye shape has its own individual characteristics, changing our goals each time.

hooded eyes

Hooded eyes are sometimes called "bedroom eyes" because the lids tend to look partly closed and heavy. There are two types of hooded eyes—the ones you're born with and the ones you acquire. Some people, based on ethnic background or natural facial features, are born with a hooded eyelid. Other people acquire hooded eyes as they age; minimizing the fullness of the lids will make you look years younger. When you look at a hooded eye, you see more eyelid than you do eye. It is full and puffy with no defined crease. The upper part of the lid lays on top of the lower part of the lid, hiding the crease and the lower portion of the top eyelid. Applied correctly, eye color can help hooded eyes appear more open by minimizing the eyelid. Our goal is to make the fleshy lid area recede and to make your eyes look more prominent than your eyelids.

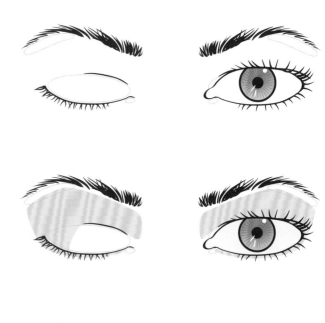

- If you have hooded eyes, you can pull off a smoky eye if you want drama. For a more natural look, creating a gradation of color from dark at the outer corner to lighter as you move across the eyelid will help open the eye up.

- Don't highlight your brow bone too much, which will accentuate the hooded appearance of your eyelid.

- Never apply your highlight shade over your entire lid (above the first fold or crease in your specific lid); it will just make it look even more hooded.

Let's look at multiple hooded eyes to get a full picture of what to do to make this eye shape look its best. The diagram above shows where to place your highlight, midtone, and contour shades.

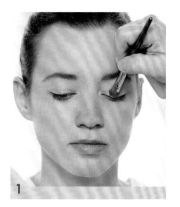

hooded eyes (born with)

1. Using a #22 highlight brush, apply a shimmery beige crème-to-powder eye shadow to your eyelid all along your lash line up to your first crease or fold, not above onto the fleshy part of the lid.

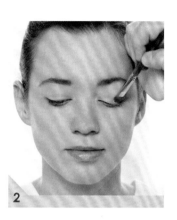

2. With the same brush, apply a powder shimmer champagne shadow directly over the crème. Layering the two will make your highlight more intense, opening the eye up. You could also highlight your brow bone; here we simply concealed and powdered it (when we prepped the eyelid).

3. Curl your eyelashes and apply the first layer of mascara to your top lashes.

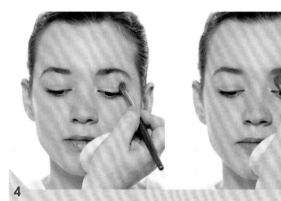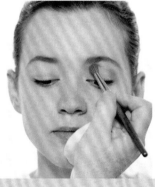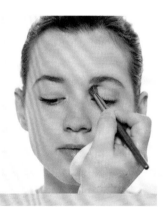

4. With a #11 midtone brush and a matte taupe eye shadow, start at the outside corner base of your upper lash line and bring the color up and over the entire hooded area. This helps the lid recede, pushing it away and bringing the eye forward. With this eye shape, you want to always use a matte midtone because you have a lot of lid to push back to visually open the eye.

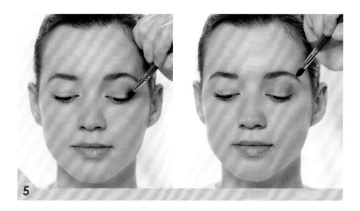

5. Using a #30 contour brush, apply your midtone to the outer corner of your eyelid to help close in the outer corner.

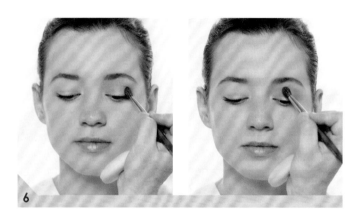

6. With a #16 blending brush (the one that is always clean and ready to blend with), blend out your midtone so there are no hard edges.

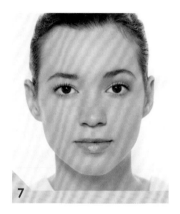

7. Compare one eye with midtone and one without; your midtone really opens the eye up. In the end, it will pretty much disappear, but it does all the heavy lifting.

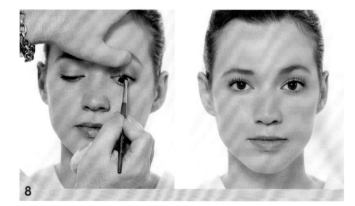

8. To start your lash line definition, using a #41 detail eye liner brush, push a matte black eye shadow into the base of your lash line. You can see here how it starts to create definition on her left eye and is making her eyelashes look thicker.

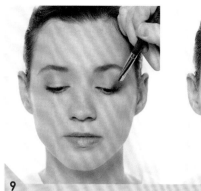

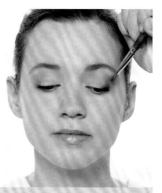

9. For more intense color and to help create a better gradation of color from dark to light, start with a crème shadow at the base of the lash line in the outer corner of the eyelid. Using another #22 highlight brush, apply a shimmery copper crème shadow.

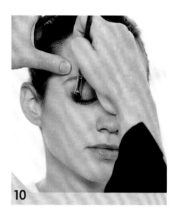

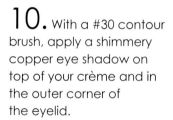

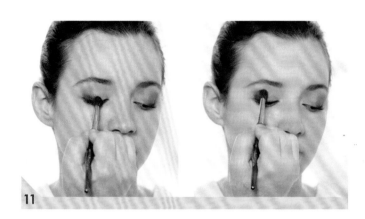

10. With a #30 contour brush, apply a shimmery copper eye shadow on top of your crème and in the outer corner of the eyelid.

11. With a #16 blending brush, start blending at the base of the lash line and bring the color up and over the hooded area, layering it on top of your midtone. Blend it up toward where the crease should be and in toward the center of the lid. Bring your contour color in a little more and up a little higher than you did on the basic eye. Don't bring it as far across as you did your mid-tone, but come halfway across the lid. This will help the hooded area recede.

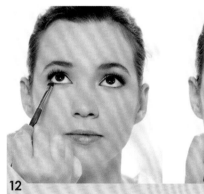

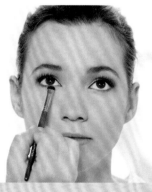

12. Using a #38 detail eye shadow brush, apply your midtone along your lower lash line, starting from the outside corner and brushing across toward the inside corner; this helps start your definition and create a better blend when you apply your contour shade and eyeliner.

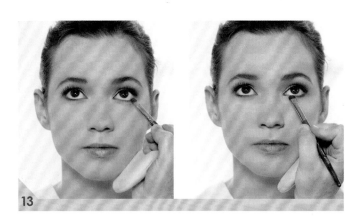

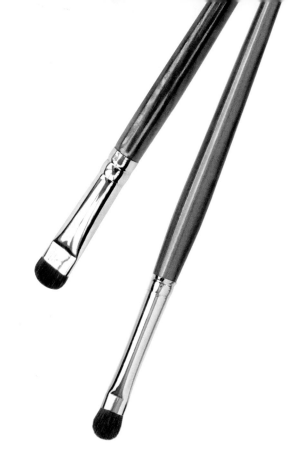

13. With the same brush, sweep your contour color underneath the bottom lashes to define the lower lash line, starting from the outside corner and blending your way across. You don't want to miss this step! Hooded eyes really benefit from a well-defined upper and lower lash line.

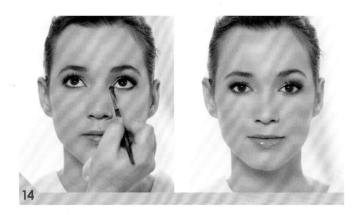

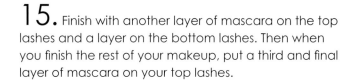

14. With a #14 detail eye shadow brush, apply your highlight shadow to the inside corner of the lower lash line. This will really help open up your eyes, making them appear larger.

15. Finish with another layer of mascara on the top lashes and a layer on the bottom lashes. Then when you finish the rest of your makeup, put a third and final layer of mascara on your top lashes.

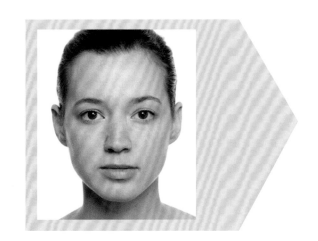

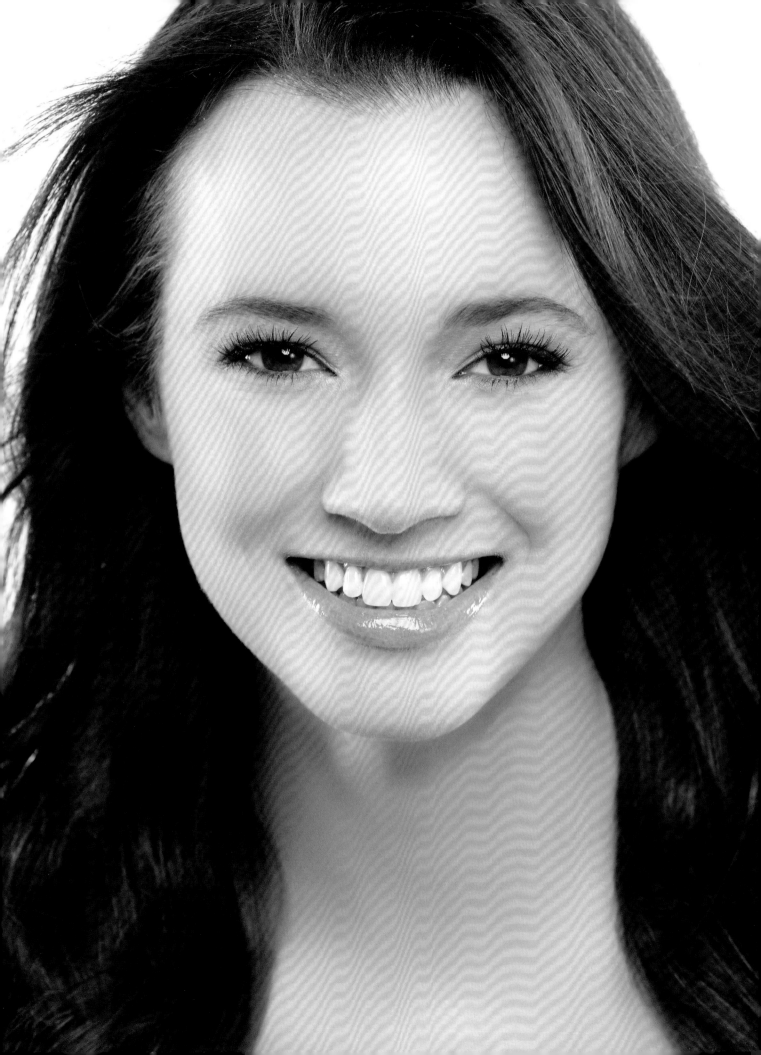

hooded eye (acquired)

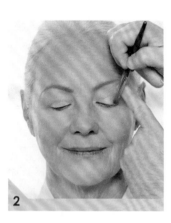

1. Using a #14 detail eye shadow brush, apply a shimmery beige crème-to-powder eye shadow to your eyelid all along your lash line up to your first crease or fold, not above onto the fleshy part of the lid, which in this case is quite close to the lash line.

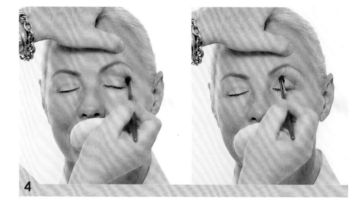

2. With a #22 highlight brush, apply a powder shimmer champagne shadow directly over the crème. Layering the two will make your highlight more intense, opening the eye up. You could also highlight your brow bone; here we simply concealed and powdered it (when we prepped the eyelid).

3. Curl your eyelashes and apply the first layer of mascara to your top lashes.

4. With a #27 midtone brush and a matte taupe eye shadow, start at the outside corner base of your upper lash line and bring the color up and over the entire hooded area. This helps the lid recede, pushing it away and bringing the eye forward. With this eye shape, you want to always use a matte midtone because you have a lot of lid to push back to visually open the eye.

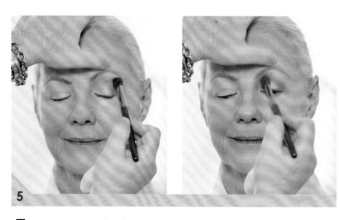

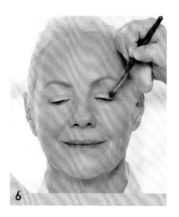

5. With a #28 blending brush (the one that is always clean and ready to blend with), blend out your midtone so there are no hard edges.

6. Using a #30 contour brush, apply your midtone to the outer corner of your eyelid to help close in the outer corner.

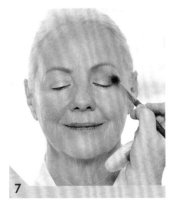
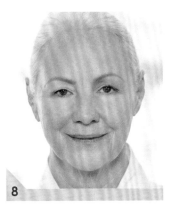
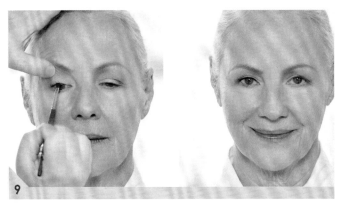

7. Blend the area again, this time with a #16 blending brush.

8. Compare one eye with midtone and one eye without; your midtone really opens the eye up. In the end, it will pretty much disappear, but it does all the heavy lifting.

9. To start your lash line definition, using a #41 detail eye liner brush, push a matte black eye shadow into the base of your lash line.

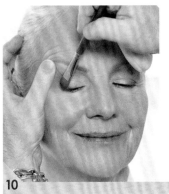
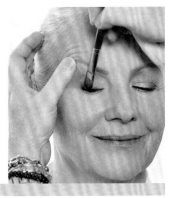
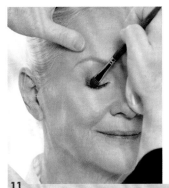
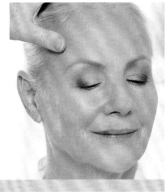

10. For more intense color and to help create a better gradation of color from dark to light, start with a crème shadow at the base of the lash line in the outer corner of the eyelid. Using another #22 highlight brush, apply a shimmery copper crème shadow.

11. With a #30 contour brush, apply a shimmery copper eye shadow right on top of your crème and in the outer corner of the eyelid.

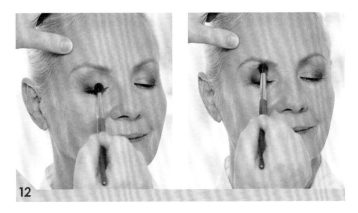

12. With a #16 blending brush, start blending at the base of the lash line and bring the color up and over the hooded area, layering it on top of your midtone. Blend it up toward where the crease should be and in toward the center of the lid. Bring your contour color in a little more and up a little higher than you did on the basic eye. Don't bring it as far across as you did your midtone, but come halfway across the lid. This will help the hooded area recede.

13. To create more definition at the lash line (which is always great for a hooded eye), line your eyes with a black eyeliner right along the lash line, keeping the line as close to the lash line as possible. Make sure it is the thinnest at the inside corner, slowly getting thicker as you get to the outside corner.

14. For the perfect amount of drama, apply false eyelashes (see page 188).

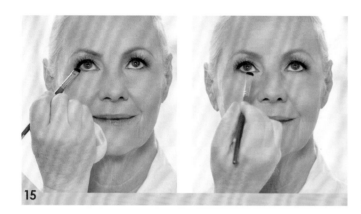

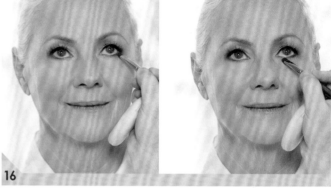

15. Using a #38 detail eye shadow brush, apply your midtone along your lower lash line, starting from the outside corner and brushing across toward the inside corner; this helps start your definition and create a better blend when you apply your contour shade and eyeliner.

16. With the same brush, sweep your contour color underneath the bottom lashes to define the lower lash line, starting from the outside corner and blending your way across. You don't want to miss this step! Hooded eyes really benefit from well-defined upper and lower lash lines.

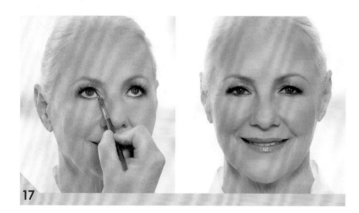

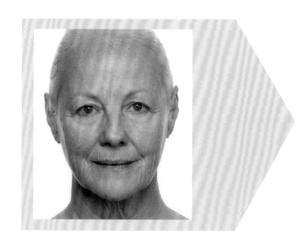

17. With a #14 detail eye shadow brush, apply your highlight shadow to the inside corner of your lower lash line. This will really help open up your eyes, making them appear larger.

18. Finish with another layer of mascara on the top lashes, blending them into your false eyelashes, and a layer on the bottom lashes.

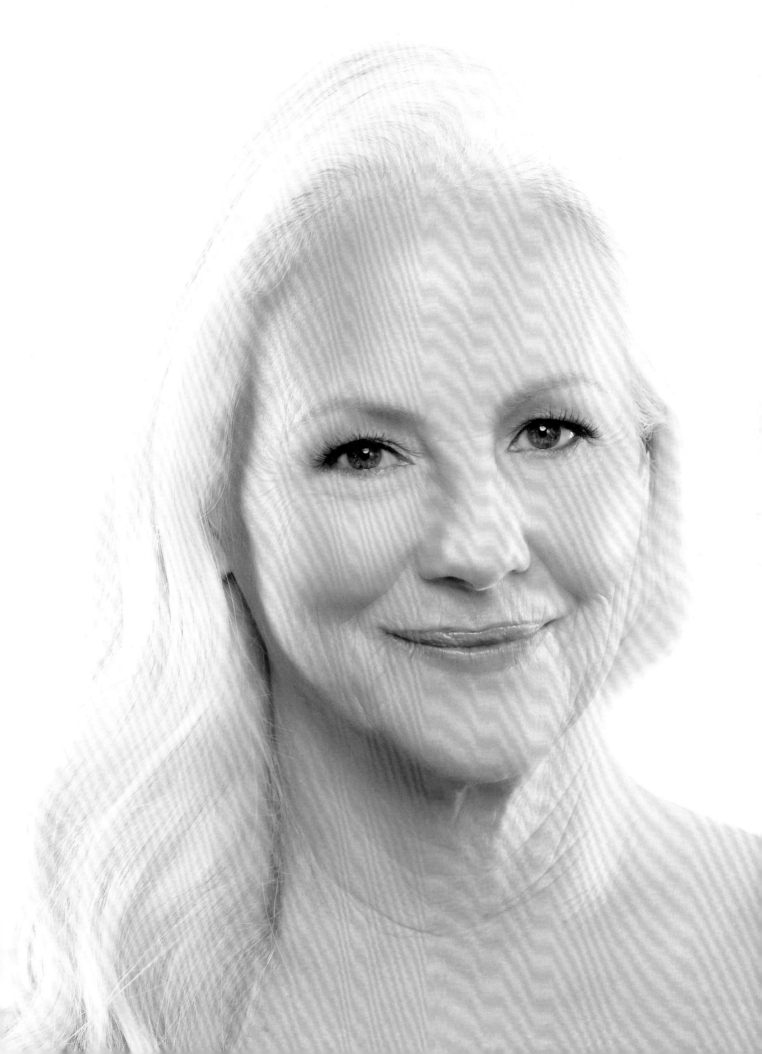

hooded eye (born with)

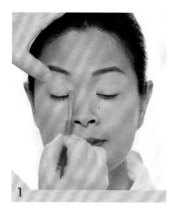

1. Some might call this hooded lid a monolid, but it is still a hooded eyelid. With this eye, we are creating the illusion of a new crease. Using a #22 highlight brush, apply a shimmery beige crème-to-powder eye shadow to your eyelid starting at the base of your lash line and bring it up to where you want to make your new crease.

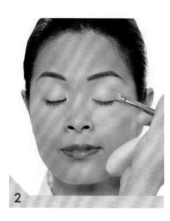

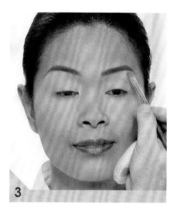

2. With the same brush, apply a layer of matte beige and a layer of shimmer champagne powder eye shadow directly over the crème. Layering the two powders will make your lid opaque. The eye shadow you touch first will be on top and the eye shadow you touch second will be against your skin.

3. With the same brush, apply the matte beige eye shadow to just your brow bone.

4. Curl your eyelashes and apply the first layer of mascara to your top lashes.

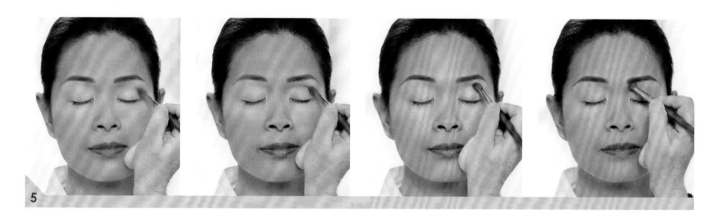

5. With a #11 midtone brush and a matte taupe midtone eye shadow, start at the outside corner of the eyelid so that area will get the most midtone color. Gently move your brush along the crease into the inside corner of the eyelid (from the outside corner all the way across to the inside corner). You're basically drawing on the crease you want to see. If you want it more defined, apply a few more layers of your midtone shade (feel free to layer for more definition).

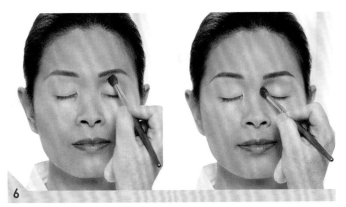

6. With a #16 blending brush (the one that is always clean and ready to blend with), blend out your midtone so there are no hard edges.

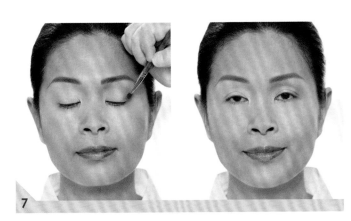

7. Using a #30 contour brush, apply your midtone to the outer corner of your eyelid, to help close in the outer corner.

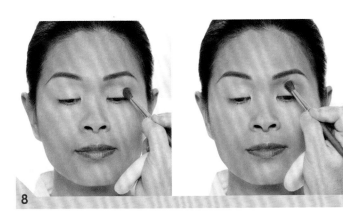

8. Blend with a #16 blending brush.

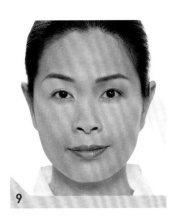

9. Compare one eye with midtone and one without; your midtone really opens the eye up and creates the illusion of a lid and a crease. In the end, it will pretty much disappear, but it does all the heavy lifting.

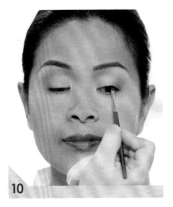

10. To start your lash line definition, using a #41 detail eye liner brush, push a matte black eye shadow into the base of your lash line.

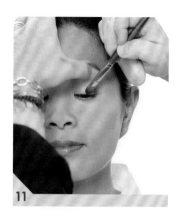

11. For more intense color and to help create a better gradation of color from dark to light, start with a crème shadow at the base of the lash line in the outer corner of the eyelid. Using another #22 highlight brush, apply a shimmery copper crème shadow.

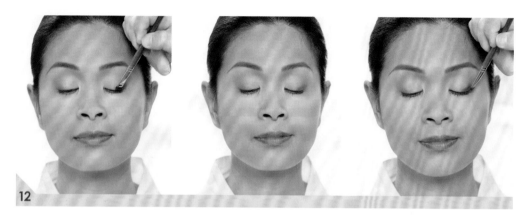

12. With a #38 detail eye shadow brush, apply a shimmery brown eye shadow right on top of your crème and in the outer corner of the eyelid.

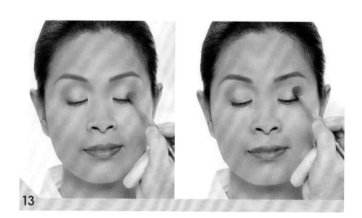

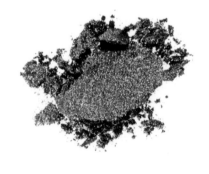

13. With a #16 blending brush, start blending at the base of the lash line and bring the color up and over the hooded area, layering it on top of your midtone. Blend it up toward where the crease should be and in toward the center of the lid. Bring your contour color in a little more and up a little higher than you did on the basic eye. Don't bring it as far across as you did your midtone, but come halfway across the lid. This will help the hooded area recede.

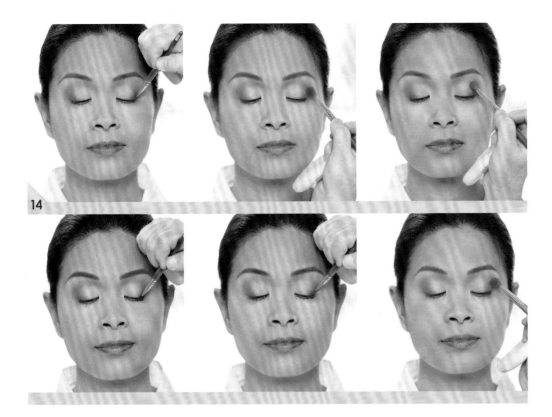

14. Keep layering until you get the depth and shaping you want.

15. To create more definition at the lash line (which is always great for a hooded eye), line your eyes with a black eyeliner right along the lash line, keeping the line as close to the lash line as possible. Make sure it is thinnest at the inside corner, slowly getting thicker as you get to the outside corner.

16. For the perfect amount of drama, apply false eyelashes (see page 188).

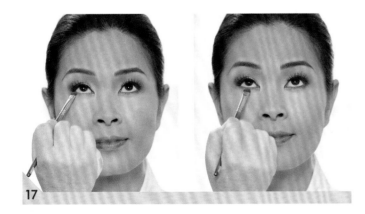

17. Using a #38 detail eye shadow brush, apply your midtone along your lower lash line, starting from the outside corner and brushing across toward the inside corner; this helps start your definition and create a better blend when you apply your contour shade and eyeliner.

tip: *Your eyebrow shape is very important here because attention can be diverted from the hooded eyelid with a beautifully shaped eyebrow.*

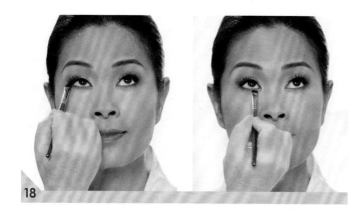

18. With the same brush, sweep your contour color underneath the bottom lashes to define the lower lash line, starting from the outside corner and blending your way across. You don't want to miss this step! Hooded eyes really benefit from well-defined upper and lower lash lines.

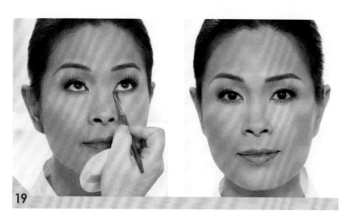

19. With a #14 detail eye shadow brush, apply your highlight shadow to the inside corner of your lower lash line. This will really help open up your eyes, making them appear larger.

20. Finish with another layer of mascara on the top lashes, blending them into your false eyelashes, and a layer on the bottom lashes.

tip: *With this eye shape, you must curl your eyelashes! It will help push the lid back and open up your eye.*

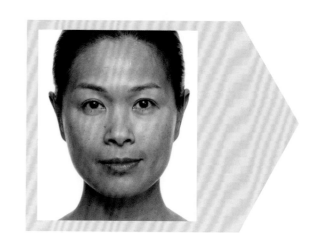

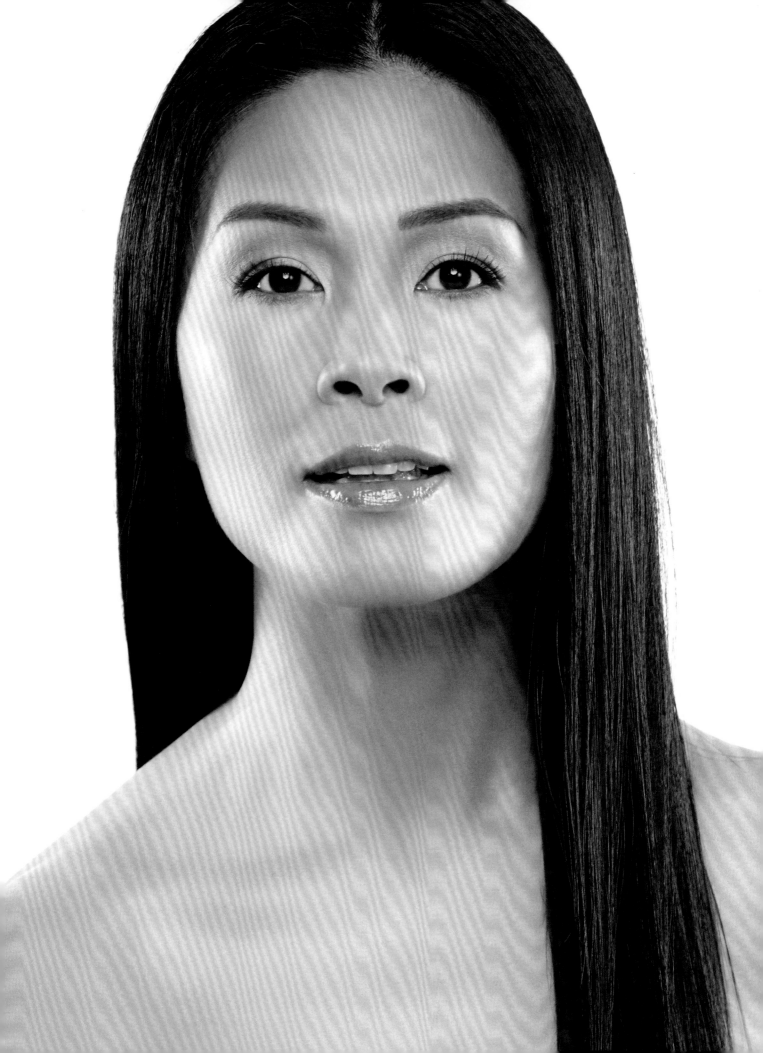

deep-set eyes

Deep-set eyes are set deep into their sockets, and the brow bone extends out farther than it does with any other eye shape. The goal with deep-set eyes is to bring your eyes out and forward, while pushing your brow bone back. Achieving this will make your eyes look more properly set on your face. The great thing about deep-set eyes is that they are much less likely to start to droop as you age. Here's what you need to know:

- A dark eyelid does not work with this eye shape. You want to highlight the eyelids of deep-set eyes as much as possible to help bring them out. A dark lid will just push them farther back.

- Darkening the crease is also unnecessary for this eye shape.

- There is no need to highlight your brow bone, because it is already prominent. Highlighting would just bring it forward even more.

- When you wear eyeliner on this eye shape, keep it very thin and as close to the lash line as possible. Thick eyeliner will work against you when you're trying to bring the eyes out, especially on the upper lids.

This diagram below shows where to add your highlight, midtone, and contour shades.

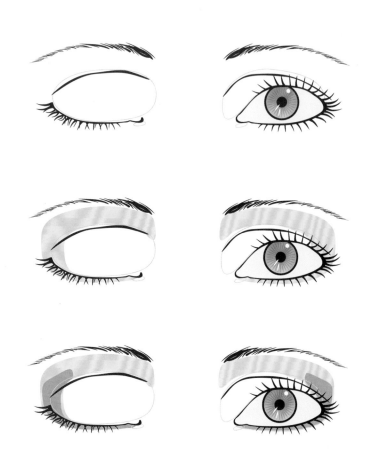

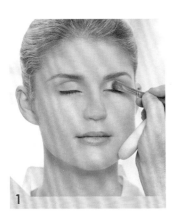

1. Using a #22 highlight brush, apply a shimmery beige crème-to-powder eye shadow to your eyelid and up into the crease. This really helps pull the eye forward.

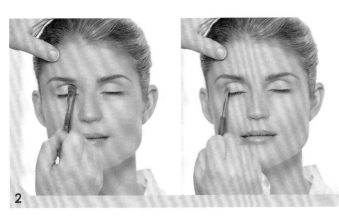

2. With the same brush, layer a matte beige eye shadow and a shimmery champagne eye shadow on top of your crème. Remember, when you load your brush, what you touch first will be on top and what you touch second will be next to your skin. You want this lid to be nice and shimmery. Layering will give you the shimmer you need along with a great opaque coverage.

3. Curl your eyelashes and apply the first layer of mascara to your top lashes.

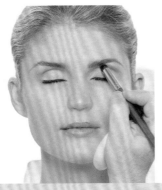

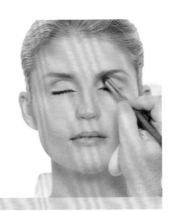

4. With a #20 ultimate crease brush for great control, apply a matte taupe midtone eye shadow right above the crease, not in it. Starting from the outside corner, bring it across the lid toward the inside corner just above the crease.

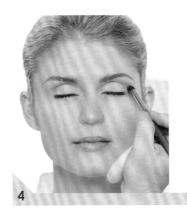

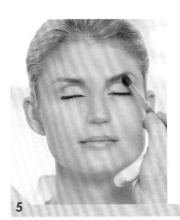

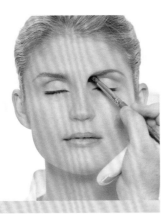

5. Using a #16 blending brush (the one that is always clean and ready to blend with), blend up toward the brow bone—not all the way to the brow, but toward the brow. Deepening the brow bone will visually push the brow bone away from us. So, by highlighting your lid, we have brought it forward, and by deepening your brow bone, we have pushed it away from us, making your eye look more properly set on your face.

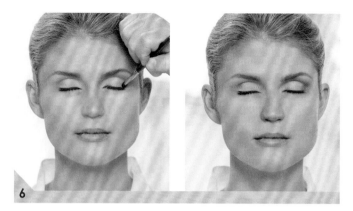

6. Using a #30 contour brush, apply your midtone to the outer corner of your eyelid to help close in the outer corner.

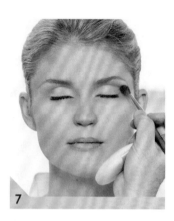

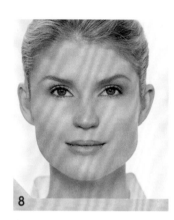

7. Blend with a #16 blending brush.

8. As you can see, the highlight and the midtone really start to put the eye back in the right place. We could line and add eyelashes and have a nice polished eye at this point. Your midtone does so much for correcting your eye placement. In the end, it will pretty much disappear, but it does all the heavy lifting.

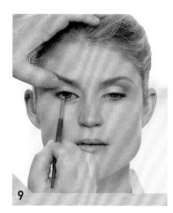

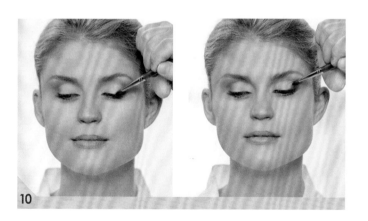

9. To start the lash line definition, use a #41 detail eye liner brush to push a matte black shadow into the base of your lash line.

10. For more intense color and to help create a better gradation of color from dark to light, start with a crème shadow at the base of the lash line in the outer corner of the eyelid. Using another #22 highlight brush, apply a shimmery copper crème shadow.

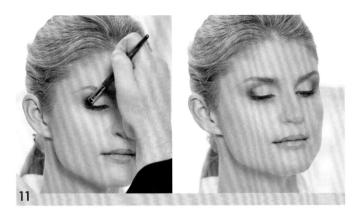

11. Using a #38 detail eye shadow brush so you'll have great control, apply a shimmery copper shadow directly on top of the crème you just applied.

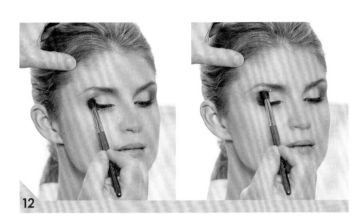

12. Use a #16 blending brush to blend into the outer corner of the eyelid and up onto the brow bone to help push the area away (make it recede). Be careful to keep the blending tight and controlled; you don't want to darken the eyelid too much, which would push the eye back into the head.

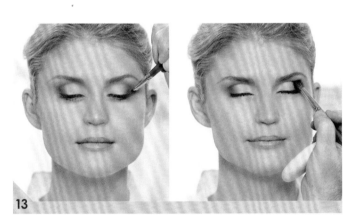

13. Keep layering until you get the intensity you want.

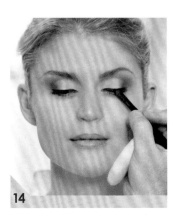

14. To create more definition at the lash line, line your eyes with a black eyeliner right along the lash line, keeping the line as close to your lash line as possible so you don't darken the lid. Make sure it is thinnest at the inside corner, slowly getting thicker as you get to the outside corner.

15. For the perfect amount of drama, apply false eyelashes (see page 188).

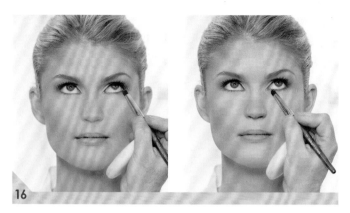

16. Using a #13 detail eye shadow brush, apply your midtone along your lower lash line, starting from the outside corner and brushing across toward the inside corner. This helps start your definition and creates a better blend when you apply your contour shade and if you choose to use eyeliner.

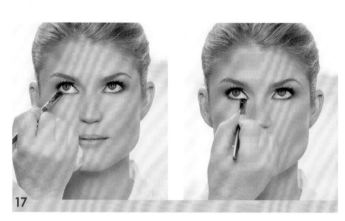

17. With a #38 detail eye shadow brush, sweep the contour color underneath your bottom lashes to define the lower lash line, starting from the outside corner and blending your way across.

18. With a #14 detail eye shadow brush, apply your highlight shadow to the inside corner of your lower lash line. This will really help open up your eyes, making them appear larger.

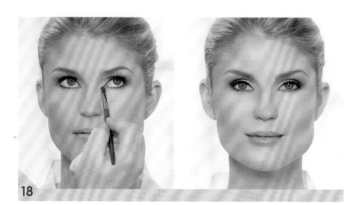

19. Finish with another layer of mascara on your top lashes, blending them into your false eyelashes, and a layer on the bottom lashes.

tip: *For drama, I always use a brighter (not necessarily a darker) contour shadow. This way, you do not deepen your lid too much.*

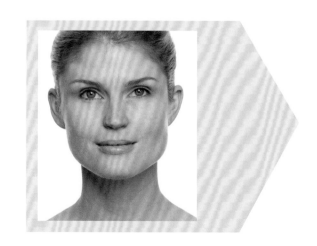

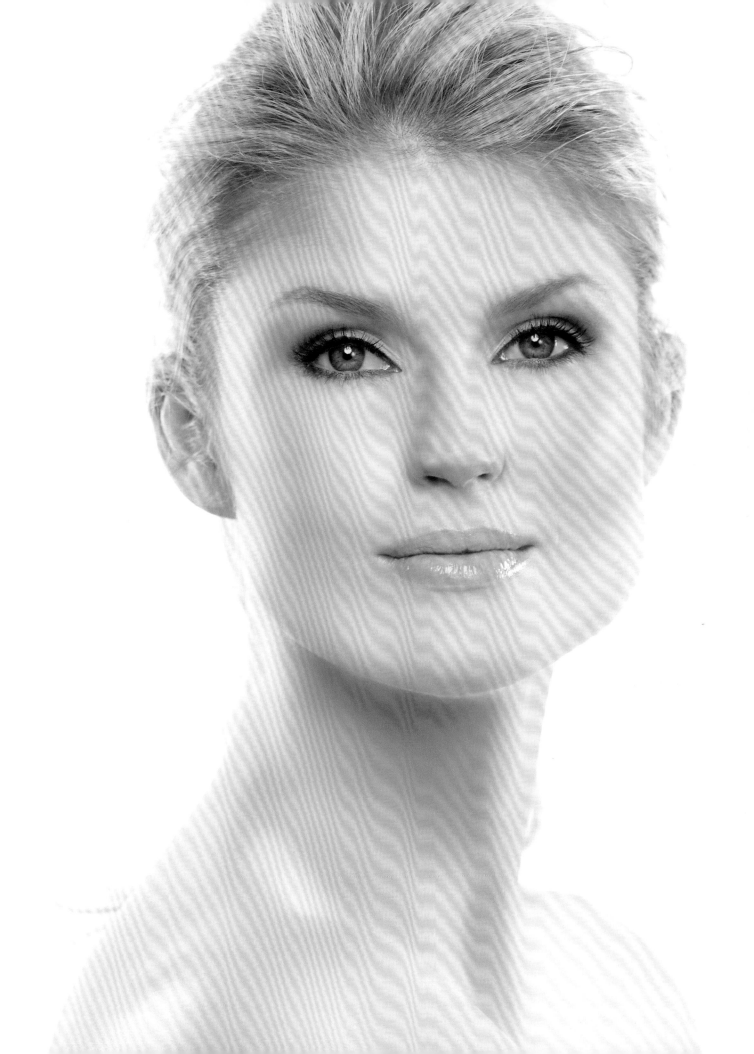

close-set eyes

The ideal space between your eyes is approximately the width of one eye. If your eyes are spaced any closer than that, you have close-set eyes. Your goal is to create the illusion of eyes that are placed farther apart. Here's what you need to know:

- Keep the inside corners of your eyes and the areas closest to your nose as light as possible to help visually "push" the eyes apart.

- Make sure to concentrate the darker shades on the outer corners of this eye shape. Elongate your darkest shadows out to help pull the eyes apart.

This diagram shows where to add your highlight, midtone, and contour shades.

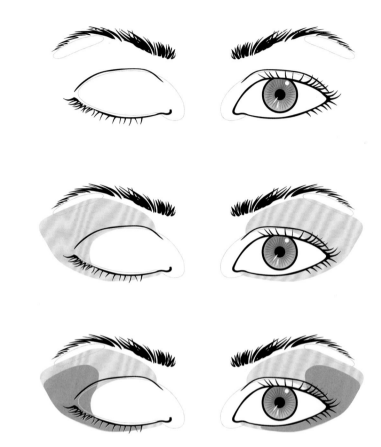

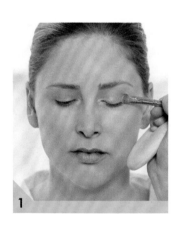

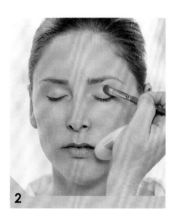

1. Using a #22 highlight brush, apply a shimmery beige crème-to-powder eye shadow to your eyelid from your lash line all the way to your crease. You are going to layer crème and powder shadow to make your lid look more dramatic.

2. With the same brush, apply a shimmery champagne eye shadow directly on top of the crème. You could apply it to your brow bone if you want to. We opted not to here; the eyelid prep was enough.

3. Curl your eyelashes and apply the first layer of mascara to your top lashes (see page 136).

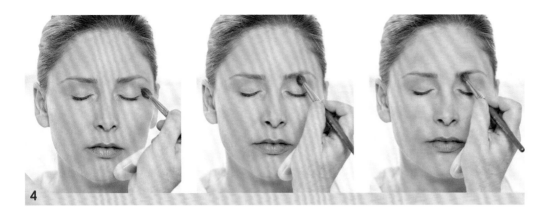

4. With a #11 midtone brush and a matte taupe eye shadow, starting at the outer corner of the crease, bring the color in toward the inside corner. With all other eye shapes, we have applied our midtone all the way across from the outer corner of the crease to the inside corner, but with close-set eyes, we will only bring it three-quarters of the way across because we do not want to deepen the inside corner of the lid. This would only visually push the eyes closer together.

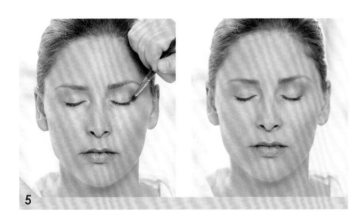

5. With a #30 contour brush, apply your midtone to the outer corner of your eyelid to help close in the outer corner.

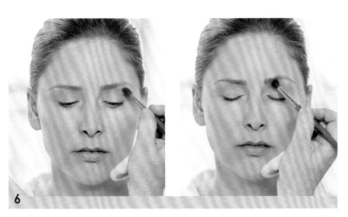

6. With a #16 blending brush (the one that is always clean and ready to blend with), blend out your midtone so there are no hard edges.

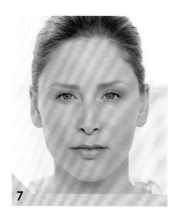

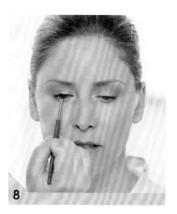

7. Compare one eye with midtone and one without; the midtone does so much to visually pull the eyes apart. In the end, it will pretty much disappear, but it does all the heavy lifting.

8. To start your lash line definition, use a #41 detail eye liner brush to push a matte black shadow into the base of your lash line.

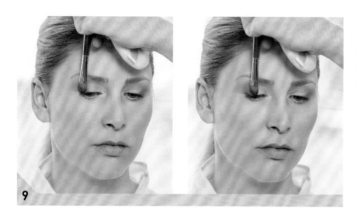

9. For more intense color and to help create a better gradation of color from dark to light, start with a crème shadow at the base of your lash line in the outer corner of your eyelid. Using another #22 highlight brush, apply a shimmery copper crème shadow.

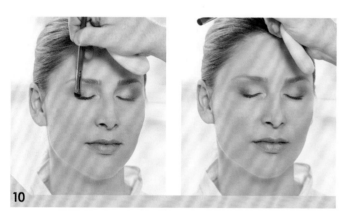

10. With a #30 contour brush, layer a shimmery brown power eye shadow directly onto your crème.

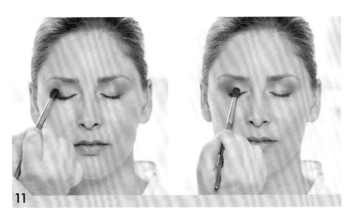

11. With a #16 blending brush, blend it across the base of your upper lash line and up into the outer area of the crease. This is the shade you want to elongate out to help pull your eyes apart visually. Confine it to the outer corners of the eyes—never bring it more than a third of the way in.

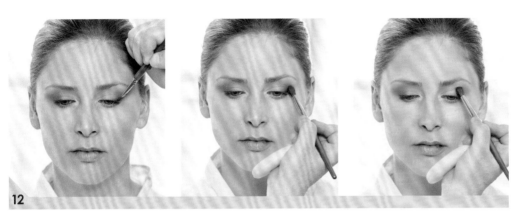

12. Keep layering until you get the depth you want.

13. To create more definition at the lash line, line your eyes with a black eyeliner right along your lash line, keeping the line as close to the lash line as possible. Make sure it is the thinnest at the inside corner, slowly getting thicker as you get to the outside corner.

14. For the perfect amount of drama, apply false eyelashes (see page 188).

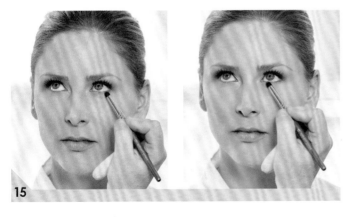

15. Using a #13 detail eye shadow brush, apply your midtone along your lower lash line, starting from the outside corner and brushing across toward the inside corner. This helps start your definition and creates a better blend when you apply your contour shade and if you choose to use eyeliner.

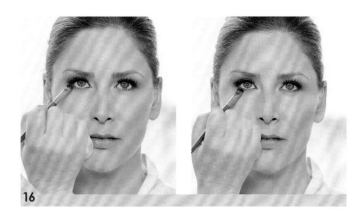

16. With a #38 detail eye shadow brush, sweep the contour color underneath your bottom lashes to define the lower lash line, starting from the outside corner and blending your way across.

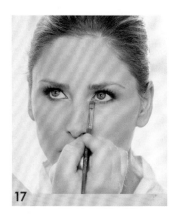

17. With a #14 detailed shadow brush, apply your highlight shadow to the inside corner of the lower lash line, making sure it wraps completely around the inside corner. For this eye shape, it not only helps open the eye up, but it is imperative in visually pushing the eyes apart.

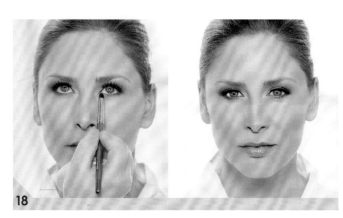

18. Make sure to blend where the highlight meets your midtone and contour.

19. Finish with another layer of mascara on the top lashes, blending them into your false eyelashes, and a layer on the bottom lashes.

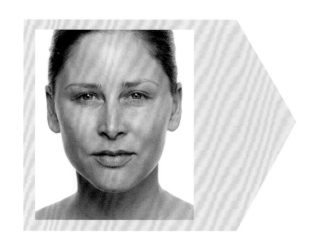

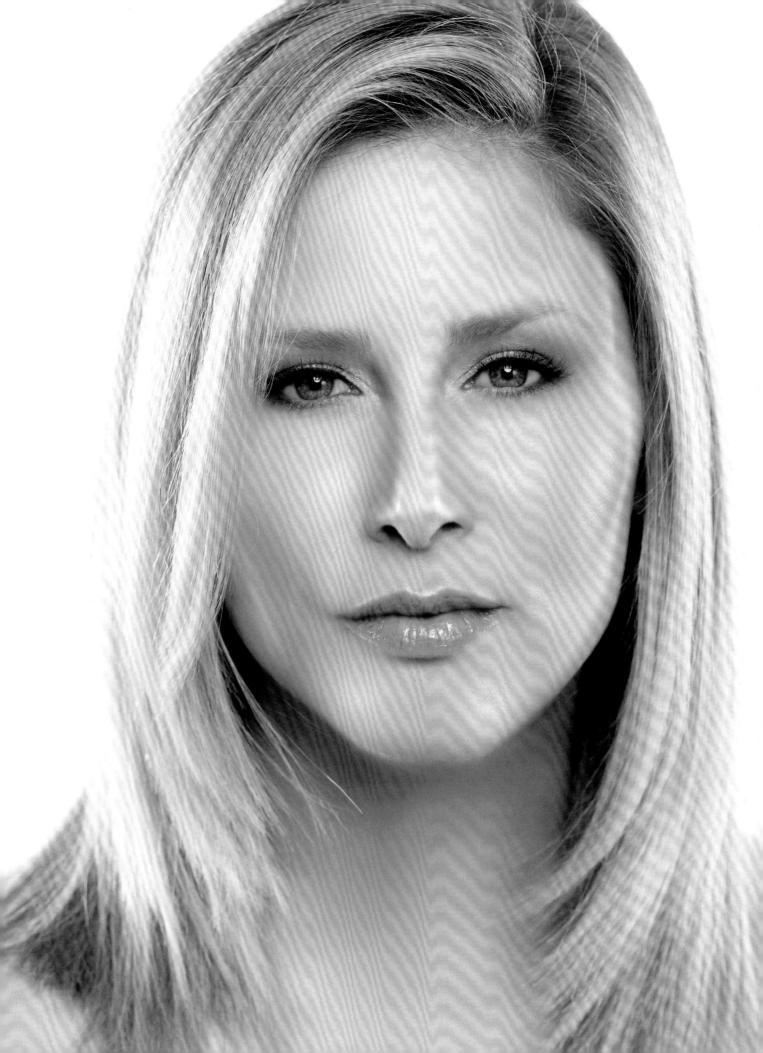

wide-set eyes

If the spacing between your eyes is wider than the width of one eye, your eyes are considered wide-set. Your goal is to create the illusion that they are set closer together (visually pushing them together). Here's what you need to know:

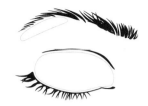

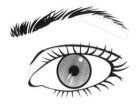

- You'll need to darken the inside hollows of your eyes, next to the bridge of your nose, more than you would for any other eye shape. Deepening the color in this area helps your eyes appear to be set closer together. To get the color depth there, do not bring your contour color all the way in—just layer your midtone to achieve the desired depth.

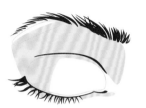

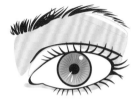

- Begin any dark-color application slightly in from the outer corner of your eye and blend your shadow up and in instead of outward because blending it outward will pull the eyes wider apart, and your goal here is to push them closer together.

This diagram shows where to add your high-light, midtone, and contour shades.

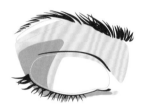

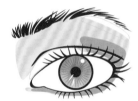

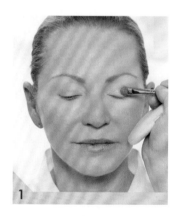

1. Using a #22 highlight brush, apply a shimmery beige crème-to-powder eye shadow to your eyelid from your lash line all the way to your crease. You are going to layer crème and powder shadow to make your lid look more dramatic.

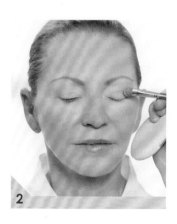

2. With the same brush, apply a shimmery champagne eye shadow directly on top of the crème. You could apply it to your brow bone if you choose. We opted not to here; the eyelid prep was enough.

3. Curl your eyelashes and apply the first layer of mascara to your top lashes (see page 136).

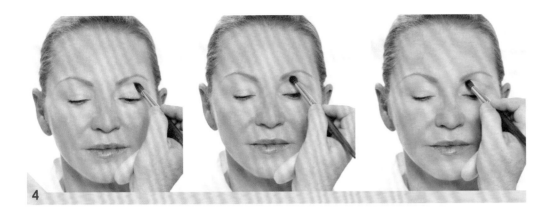

4. With a #11 midtone brush and a matte taupe eye shadow, starting from the outer corner of the crease, bring the color toward the inside corner of your eye, making sure to bring it up and in, not elongating it out. Apply a few extra layers to the inside corners to deepen the color and help visually push the eyes closer together.

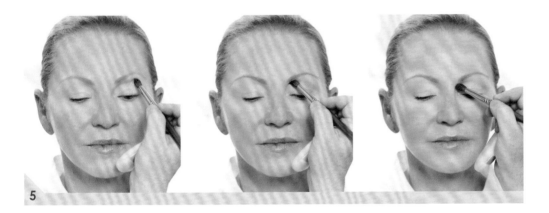

5. With a #16 blending brush (the one that is always clean and ready to blend with), blend out your midtone so there are no hard edges.

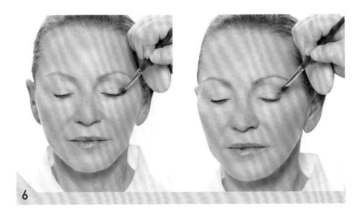

6. With a #30 contour brush, apply your midtone to the outer corner of your eyelid to help close in the outer corner.

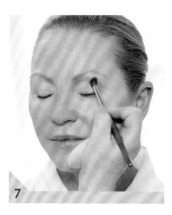

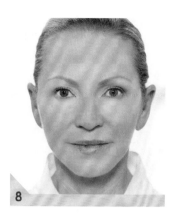

7. Using a #16 blending brush, blend the shadow you just applied.

8. Compare one eye with midtone and one without; your midtone does so much to open the eye up, define the crease, and visually push the eyes together. In the end, it will pretty much disappear, but it does all the heavy lifting.

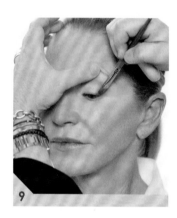

9. For more intense color and to help create a better gradation of color from dark to light, start with a crème shadow at the base of the lash line, in just slightly from the outer corner of the eyelid. Using another #22 highlight brush, apply a shimmery copper crème shadow.

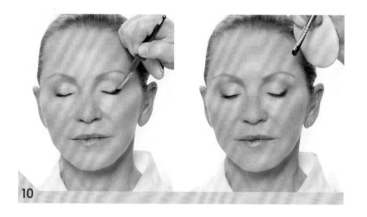

10. With a #38 detail eye shadow brush, layer a matte dark brown power eye shadow directly onto of your crème.

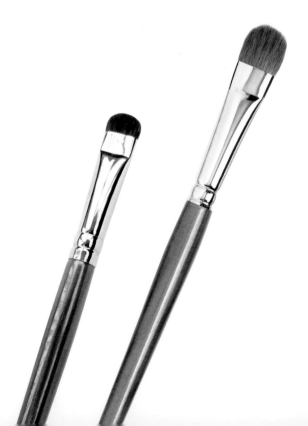

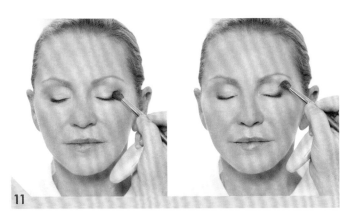

11. With a #16 blending brush, blend it across the base of your upper lash line and up into the crease. This is the shade you don't want to elongate out because it will pull the eyes apart. Remember, blend it up and in to push the eye inward.

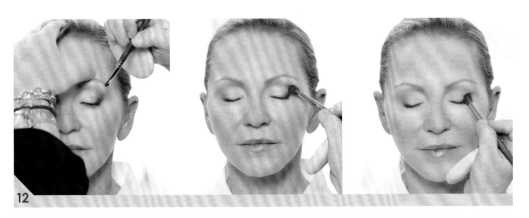

12. Keep layering until you get the level of depth you want.

13. To start the lash line definition, use a #41 detail eye liner brush to push a matte black shadow into the base of your lash line.

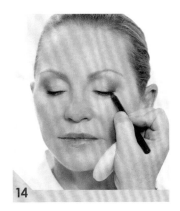

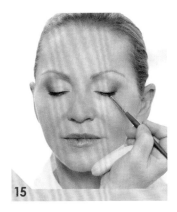

14. To create more definition at the lash line (which is always great for wide-set eyes), line your eyes with a black eyeliner right along the lash line, keeping the line as close to the lash line as possible. Make sure it is the thinnest at the inside corner, slowly getting thicker as you get to the outside corner.

15. Using a #42 eye liner brush, smooth out your liner.

16. For the perfect amount of drama, apply false eyelashes (see page 188). Start slightly in from the outside corner so you don't pull the eyes apart visually.

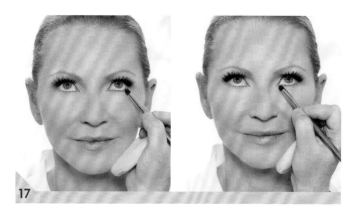

17. Using a #13 detail eye shadow brush, apply your midtone along your lower lash line, starting in just slightly from the outside corner and brushing across toward the inside corner. This helps start your definition and creates a better blend when you apply your contour shade and if you choose to use eyeliner.

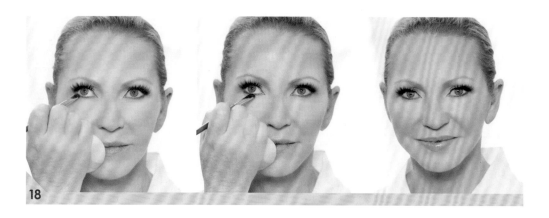

18. With a #38 detail eye shadow brush, sweep the contour color underneath your bottom lashes to define the lower lash line, starting from the outside corner and blending your way across. Be careful not to extend the color beyond the outer edge of the eye.

19. Finish with another layer of mascara on the top lashes, blending them into your false eyelashes, and a layer on the bottom lashes.

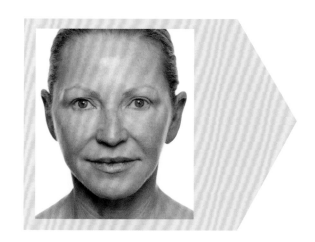

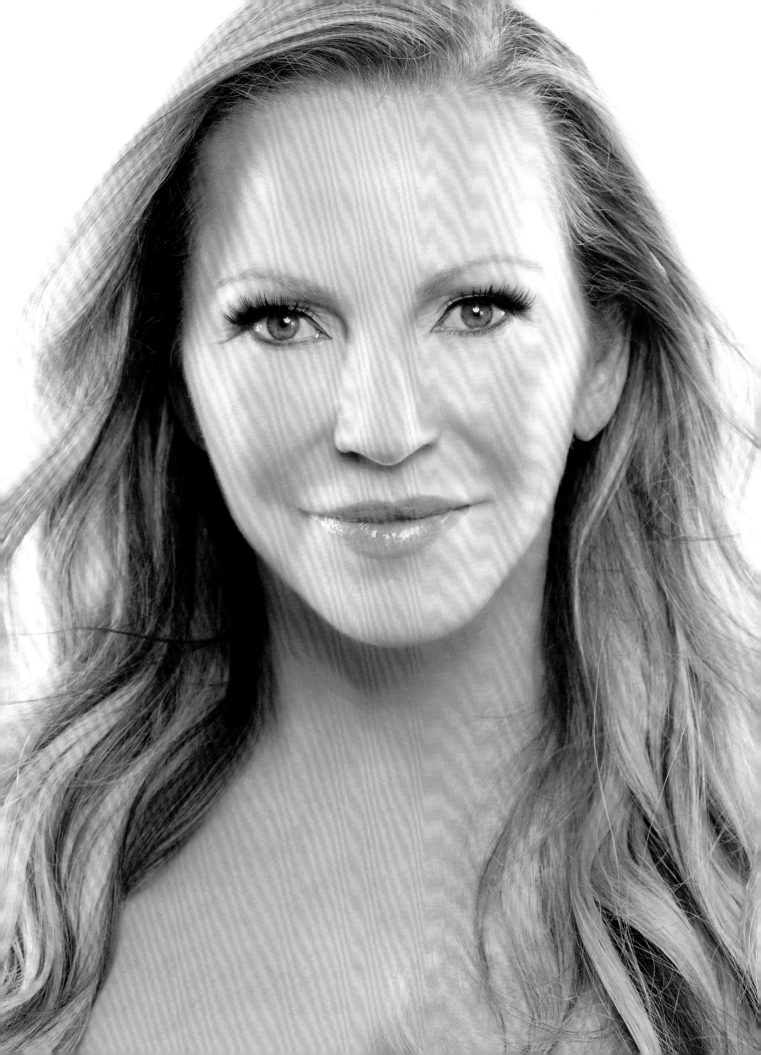

prominent eyes

If your eyelids and eyes are very full and tend to extend out from your face, you have prominent eyes. The goal here is to visually push your eye away from us and help it appear to recede more gently into your face. We do this by creating a light-to-dark effect with the three eye shadows, with the darkest shade applied closest to the lash line and fading as you go toward the brow. This is one eye shape where you are trying to make the eyes appear smaller; we want to minimize their fullness. Here's what you need to know:

- Never highlight your eyelids, or you will make your eyes appear even more prominent.

- A deeper or contour shade across the entire eyelid helps to minimize the fullness and makes it appear to recede.

- With this eye shape, you can apply your eyeliner all the way around your eye with the same thickness and intensity because we want to close the eye in slightly.

This diagram shows where to add your highlight, midtone, and contour shades.

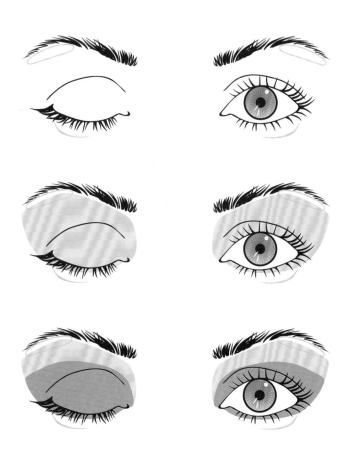

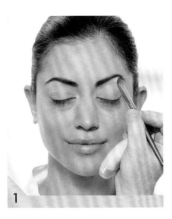

1. With a #22 highlight brush, apply a matte beige eye shadow just to your brow bone. When I say brow bone, I mean just under the arch of your brow.

2. Curl your eyelashes and apply the first layer of mascara to your top lashes (see page 136).

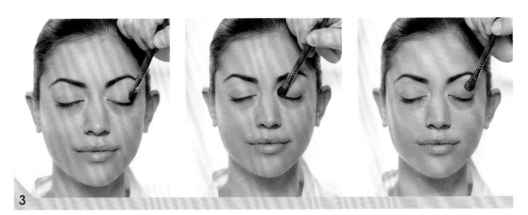

3. With a #27 eye shadow brush (because you will be applying your color to a large area), apply a matte taupe midtone eye shadow. Start at the base of your upper lash line, bring it across the lid, and then bring the color up and over your entire lid, all the way up to just under your brow bone. By starting along your lash line and working your way upward, you will get the highest concentration of color where you laid your brush first, making your color deeper at the lash line.

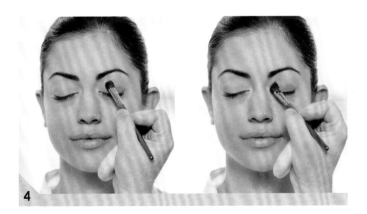

4. Using a #27 brush, apply more midtone eye shadow in a half-moon shape all along the crease to create more definition.

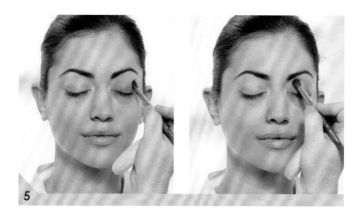

5. With a #16 blending brush (the one that is always clean and ready to blend with), blend your midtone so there are no hard edges.

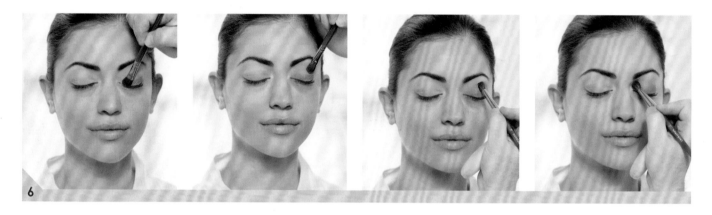

6. Keep layering until you get the desired amount of depth.

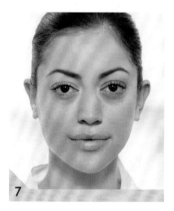

7. Compare one eye with midtone and one eye without; you can see how the midtone starts to really push the eye back into the face. In the end, it will pretty much disappear, but it does all the heavy lifting.

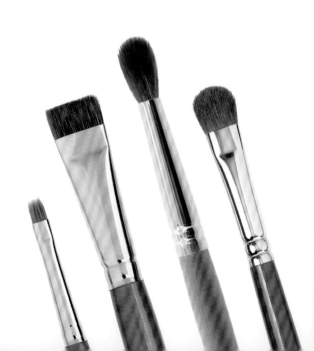

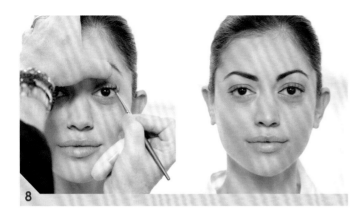

8. To start your lash line definition, use a #41 detail eye liner brush to push matte black shadow into the base of your lash line. You can see not only how it defines the lash line, but how it makes the eyelashes look thicker.

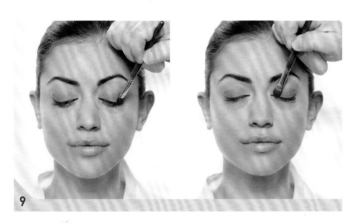

9. With a #30 contour brush and a dark shimmery brown eye shadow, start at the base of your lash line and bring the color up and over your entire lid up to your crease. This gives you the most intense color right at your lash line.

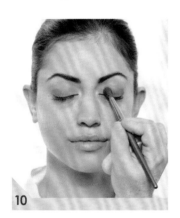

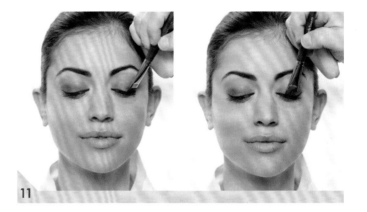

10. Blend with a #16 blending brush (the one that is always clean).

11. This eye really benefits from definition at the lash line. You could use pencil; here, I chose powder and a brush. To make it softer and look more smudged, let's use a #18 detail eye liner brush, grab some matte black shadow, and lay it all along your top lash line. As you apply it, pull up slightly with your brush to blend the line.

12. For the perfect amount of drama, apply false eyelashes (see page 188).

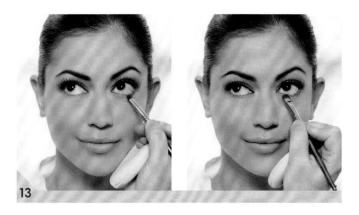

13. With a #38 detail eye shadow brush, apply your midtone shadow all along your lower lash line. Start your application from the outside corner, sweeping it across to the inside corner. This helps start your definition and creates a better blend when you apply your contour shade and if you choose to use eyeliner.

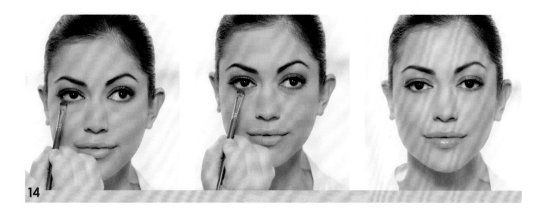

14. With the same brush, apply your contour color right over your midtone all along your lower lash line. By layering on your midtone, then your contour on top of it, you are creating a gradation color, making your lower lash line definition look more natural and blended, further helping your eyes recede into your face.

15. Finish your eyes with another layer of mascara on the top lashes, blending them into the false eyelashes, and a layer on the bottom.

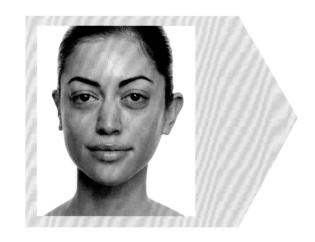

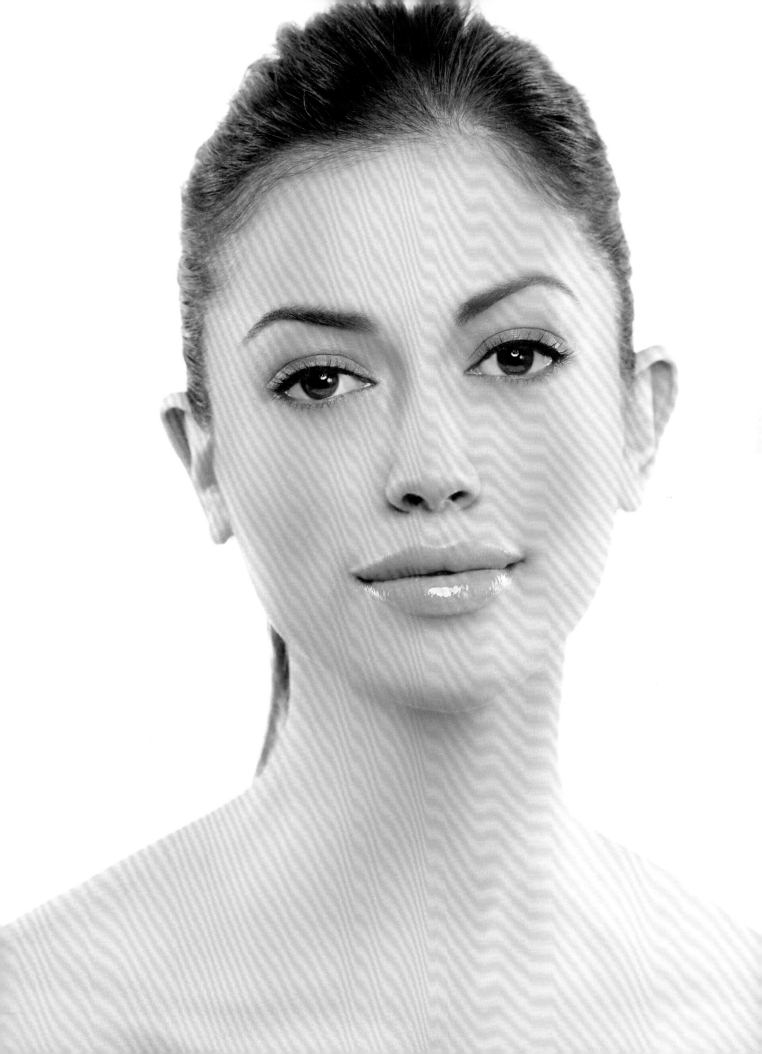

droopy eyes

When I say droopy eyes, I do not mean that the lids are droopy; I mean that the outer corners of your eyes turn slightly downward. They are sometimes referred to as "sad puppy dog eyes." Your goal is to make the outer corners appear as if they turn up rather than down. It's actually very easy to do! We just want to start all our color application in just slightly from the outside corner, on top and especially along the bottom lash line. Here's what you need to know:

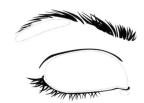 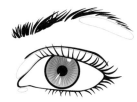

- You want to do what we call an open-ended eye, which means that the color from your top lash line and bottom lash line do not meet in the outer corner of the eye. If the color met in the outside corner, it would just accentuate the droop. By leaving it naked, you create a visual lift to the eye.

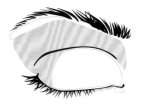 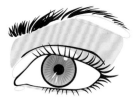

- When applying mascara, be sure to concentrate on the middle to inside lashes. Defined eyelashes in the outer corners of the eyes accentuate the droopiness.

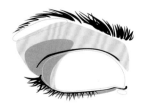 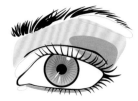

This diagram shows where to add your highlight, midtone, and contour shades.

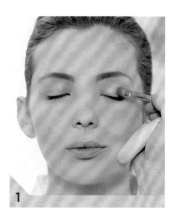

1. Using a #22 highlight brush, apply a shimmery beige crème-to-powder eye shadow to your eyelid from your lash line all the way to your crease. You are going to layer crème and powder shadow to make your lid look more dramatic.

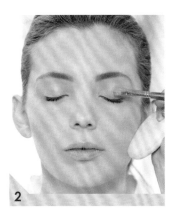

2. With the same brush, apply a shimmery champagne eye shadow directly on top of the crème. You could apply it to your brow bone if you choose. We opted not to here; the eyelid prep was enough.

3. Curl your eyelashes and apply the first layer of mascara to your top lashes (see page 136).

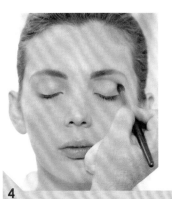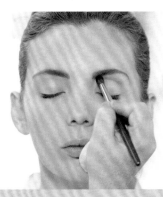

4. With a #11 midtone brush and a matte taupe midtone eye shadow, start slightly in from the outside corner so you create the illusion that the outer corner is lifted. Gently move your brush along the crease into the inside corner of the eyelid (from the outside corner all the way across to the inside corner). If you want a very defined crease, you can apply a few more layers of your midtone shade (feel free to layer for more definition).

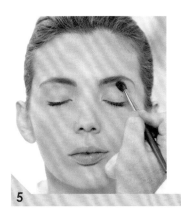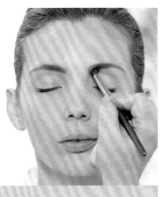

5. With a #16 blending brush (the one that is always clean and ready to blend with), smooth out your midtone so there are no hard edges.

6. To start the lash line definition, use a #41 detail eye liner brush to push a matte black shadow into the base of your lash line.

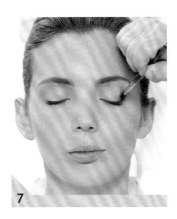

7. Using a #30 contour brush, apply more of your midtone to the outer corner of your eyelid to close it in, again slightly in from the complete outside corner to create the illusion of lift.

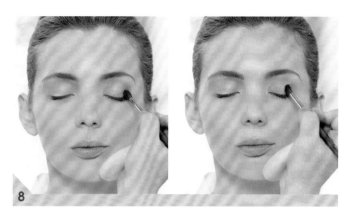

8. Use a #16 blending brush to blend the shadow you just applied.

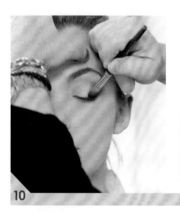
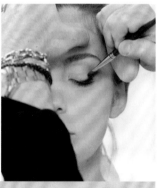

9. You can see, with just midtone on, how much shaping just your midtone does. It has already started to lift the outer corner. In the end, it will prety much disappear, but it does all the heavy lifting.

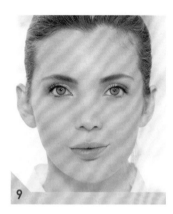

10. For more intense color and to help create a better gra dation of color from dark to light, start with a crème shadow the base of your lash line in just slightly from the outer corner the eyelid. Use another #22 highlight brush to apply a shimme copper crème shadow.

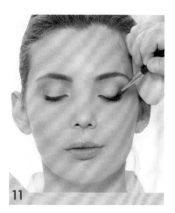

11. With a #30 contour brush, layer a shimmery copper eye shadow in the outer corner of the eyelid at the base of the lash line, on top of the crème, again in slightly from the outside corner.

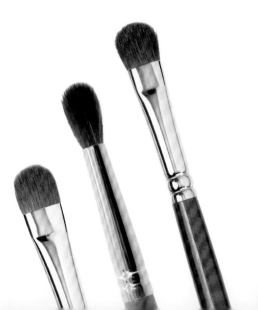

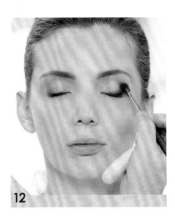

12. With a #16 blending brush (the one that is always clean and is ready to blend with), blend the color up toward the crease and in toward the inner part of the lid.

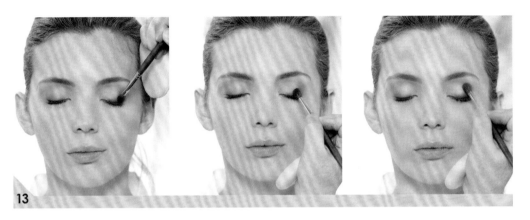

13. Keep layering on color until you reach your desired intensity with a #30 contour brush and blending it out with a #16 blending brush. Always starting just slightly in from the outside corner, bring your color up and into the crease. You can see how starting in just slightly has visually lifted the outside corner.

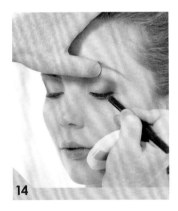

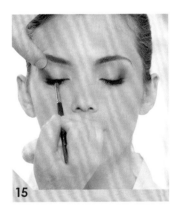

14. Using a black eyeliner, line your upper lash line (see page 130).

15. Using a #42 eye liner brush, smooth out your liner.

16. For the perfect amount of drama, apply false eyelashes (see page 188). Make sure with this eye shape to start in slightly from the outside corner so you create a visual lift.

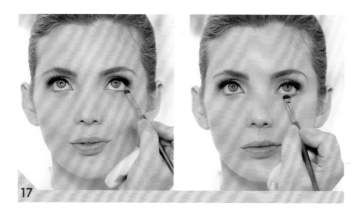

17. Using a #38 detail eye shadow brush, apply your midtone along your lower lash line, starting in just slightly from the outside corner and brushing across toward the inside corner. This helps start your definition and creates a better blend when you apply your contour shade and if you choose to use eyeliner.

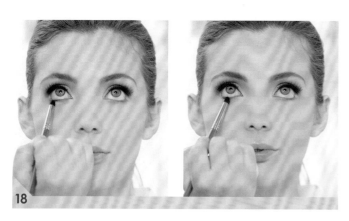

18. With a #13 detail eye shadow brush, sweep your contour color along the lower lash line, making sure once again to start slightly in from the outside corner. We don't want the color to meet at the outside corner, or it will just draw attention to the droopiness.

19. With a #14 eye shadow brush, apply your highlight shade to the inside corner of the lower lash line. This will really help open up your eyes, making them appear larger and more open.

20. Finish with another layer of mascara on the top lashes, blending them into your false eyelashes, and a layer on the bottom lashes.

tip: *With this eye shape, I would not use any eyeliner along the lower lash line. It could be too dramatic and turn your eye downward. Instead, use your contour shade to define along your lower lash line.*

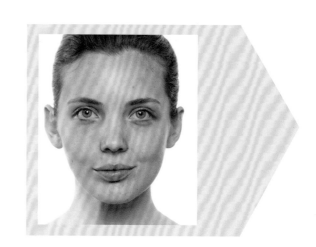

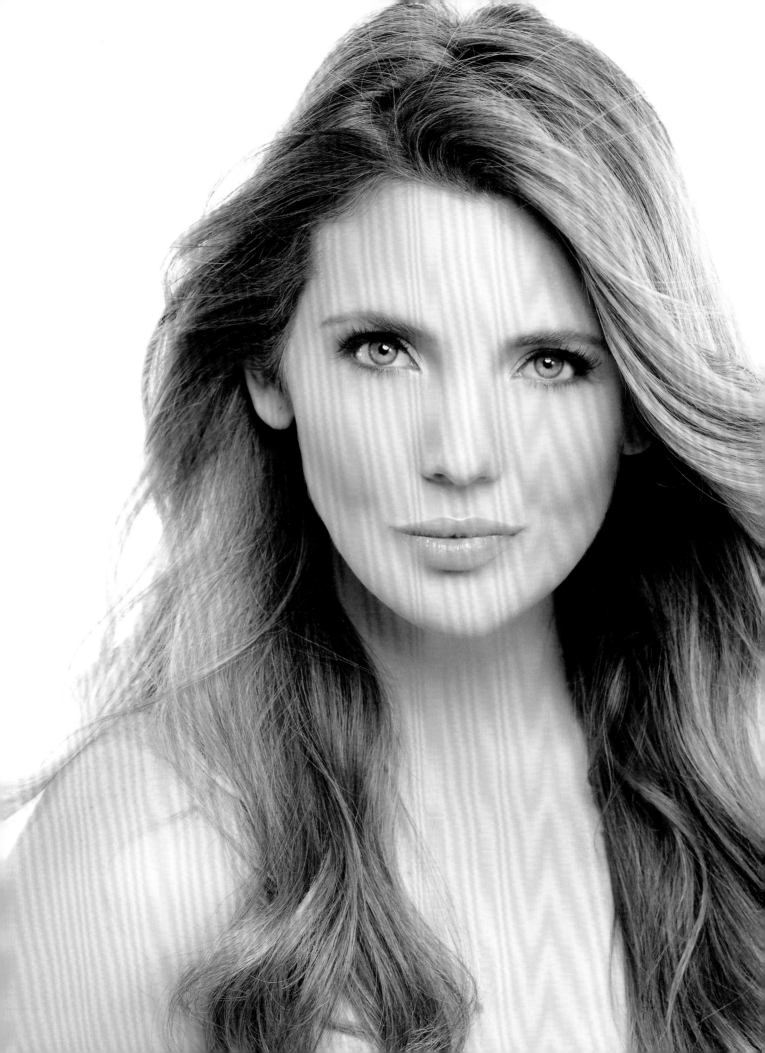

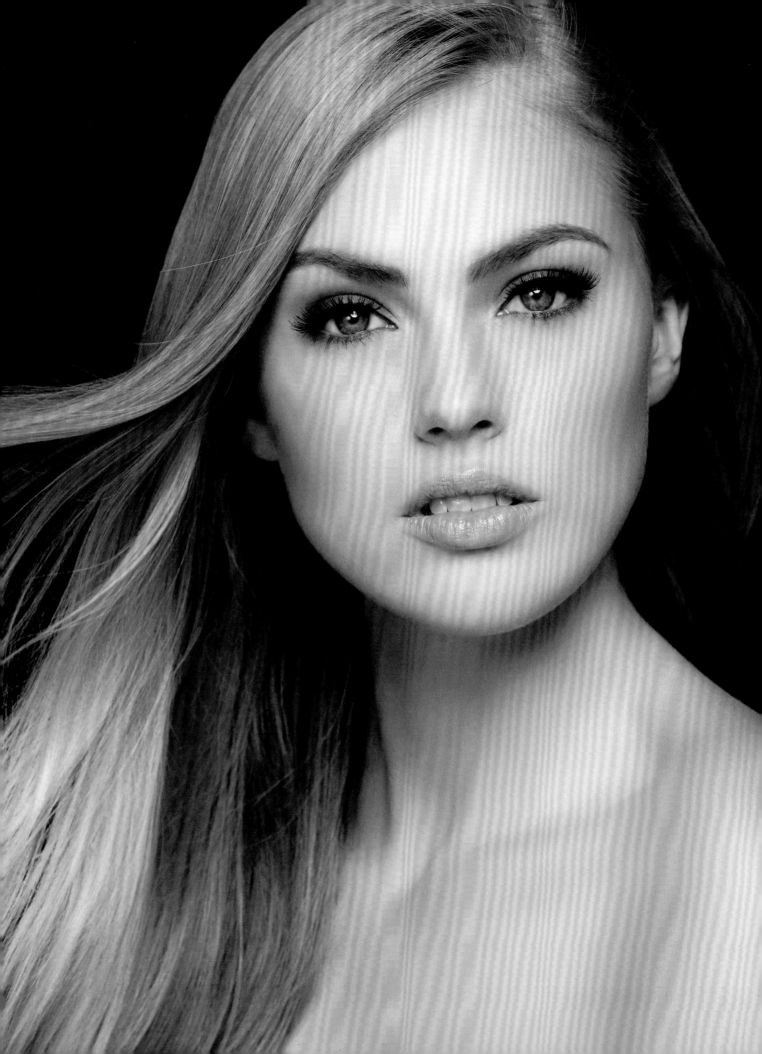

eye masterclass

As with any new artistic endeavor, once you understand the basics, you'll have the building blocks for creating any and every advanced look. Keep in mind that the impressive effects in this chapter are simply applications of basic techniques that when combined differently create something a bit more fabulous. Those tools include the most important basic components you need in creating every look, your three key eye shadows: highlight, midtone, and contour. They're your tools for being creative.

I will also be sharing some tricks and tips that will make some of the harder techniques a little easier to conquer. Most of them are classic looks with a modern twist. You will also notice that I have chosen models for some of the looks that you might not expect to see typically associated with them. I did this purposefully because I don't want you to limit who or what you think about when it comes to makeup. Be creative and explore!

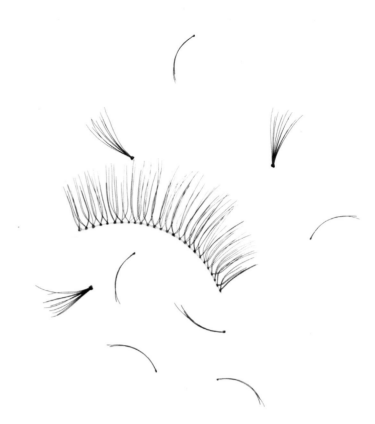

how to apply false eyelashes

Nothing takes a basic look to full glamour like a pair of false eyelashes. They are more popular than ever before, and people are wearing them all the time, even for daytime. If you want to wear them, it's important to know not only how to apply them, but how to make them look their most natural.

You have a lot choices when it comes to false eyelashes—everything from strips to individuals to flares. The most important thing to consider when it comes to strip false eyelashes is how dense they are. The denser the lash, the more likely it is to close the eye in. If you have a smaller eye, choose a lash that is wispier and more open at the base, so it helps open the eye up. If you have a larger eye, such as a prominent eye, you can pull off a denser lash because it will help close down your eye, which is your goal with your eye shape.

Next, we need to think about the band, and how it can help you achieve your end effect. If you want a more natural look, choose false eyelashes with an invisible band. If you're going for a more dramatic look, choose a strip with a black band, which will make your eye looked lined when you are finished. Lastly, I also look for a lash that is varied in length all along the perimeter; the more jagged a lash is, the more natural it will look.

Be aware that you can change the shape of your eyes with your false eyelashes. If you use a strip lash that has longer lashes in the middle, it will make your eye look rounder. If you choose a strip lash that has longer lashes at the end of the strip, it will make your eye look more elongated. They're a useful tool.

strip application

False eyelashes can seem intimidating, so here is an easy, foolproof way to apply strip false eyelashes. No matter what your makeup IQ is, this application technique will work for you and look natural:

1. Curl your natural eyelashes. If they grow straight out and down and you don't curl them, the false lash will lie straight out and down. Apply a coat of mascara; this helps keep them curled and helps the false eyelashes blend with your natural eyelashes.

2. Lay a mirror on the counter in front of you and look down. You'll be able to see everything you are about to do, and it is much more comfortable than holding your chin up so you can look into a wall mirror while everything dries.

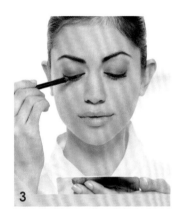
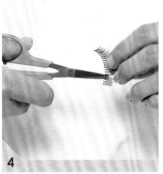
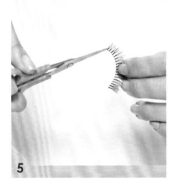
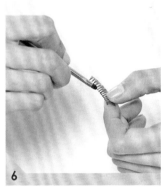

3. Draw a thin line across your upper eyelid along your lash line with a black eyeliner pencil. This is where to place the lash and conceal the lash band. Even if you don't get the false lash in place directly against your natural eyelashes, no one will know because the liner will ensure that no skin shows between your natural eyelashes and the false ones.

4. Trim the outside ends of your false eyelashes to fit the width of your eyelid. Usually, strip lashes, when used straight from their container, are too wide for most eyes. Trimming them will help them fit better and feel more comfortable. The narrower you trim them, the more comfortable and easier to apply they will be, so if you are a novice, start with narrower strips.

5. Nip the inside corners off. This will make the eyelashes more comfortable to wear. Sometimes that corner can feel like it is poking you.

6. Using liquid or gel eyeliner, color the band of your lash if it is clear/invisible. Even though it says invisible, there will be a bit of a shine to it when you are finished; coloring it black will dull that shine and make it look more natural, and it will blend into the eyeliner that you applied earlier.

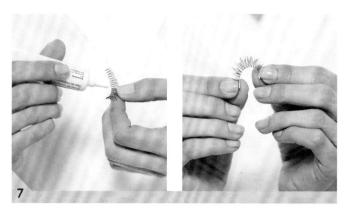

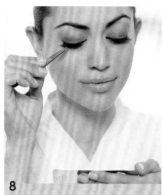

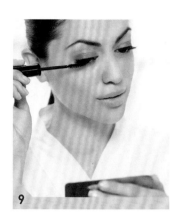

7. Apply eyelash glue to the false eyelashes all along the band. Allow the glue to dry for a minute so it gets tacky (slightly sticky). As it's drying, roll the lash so it starts to round more and takes more to the shape of your lid.

8. After you feel that the glue is tacky enough and the lash seems to have rounded, place it right on top of your eyeliner. Using the handle end of a pair of tweezers, push the lash right up against your natural lash line. Make sure to place it slightly in from the outside corner so it doesn't drag the eye down.

9. Once the glue has dried, apply a coat of mascara to blend your natural eyelashes with the false ones.

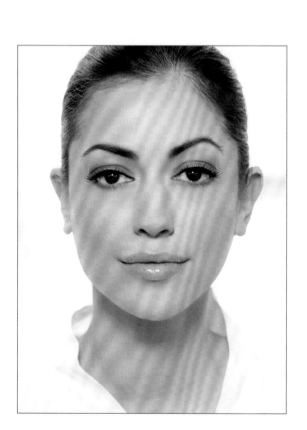

flare/strand application

Want to wear false eyelashes that look more natural than a strip? Individual flares and single strands will do just that while still demanding everyone's attention. And they're a breeze to apply:

1. Curl your natural eyelashes. If they grow straight out and down and you don't curl them, your false eyelashes will lie straight out and down too.

2. Lay a mirror on the counter in front of you and look down. You'll be able to see everything you are about to do, and it is much more comfortable than holding your chin up so you can look into a wall mirror while everything dries.

3. Apply a layer of mascara; it will give your natural eyelashes more bulk and make it easier to attach your false eyelashes.

4. Squeeze a dot of lash adhesive onto the packaging from your eyelashes. This way, you can just dip your lash into the glue. Using a pair of tweezers, grab a flare or single strand. Now dip the root end into the adhesive.

5. Lay it right on top of one of your own eyelashes, with the root of the false lash as close as possible to your natural root. Continue all across your lash line, one flare or strand at a time.

6. After the adhesive has dried, apply a coat of mascara to blend everything together.

double false eyelashes

You can create even more drama with your strip eyelashes by doubling them up. I find they look most natural when you build them on the eye rather than building them before you apply them, mainly because they form to the eye better when you build them on the eye. If you build them prior to applying them, they won't curve to the shape of your eye as well.

When applying the second lash on top of the first, make sure and set it slightly askew so the hairs fill in the gaps, creating a fuller look. You will need to cut the width a little shorter to allow you to do this. A double lash will create a denser lash, so makes sure your eye can take it.

smoky eye

One of the most searched out makeup techniques is the smoky eye. Sexy and dramatic, it's a go-to for evenings and special occasions. Done correctly, it can be stunningly gorgeous; done wrong, it can be your biggest fashion mistake. That is why it is so important to learn the most impactful way to apply it. Remember, smoky is a technique; it's about the way it's applied, not just black or super dark eye shadow. You can use any shade in a smoky application; it doesn't have to be black eye shadow to make it a smoky eye. Let's get started.

This diagram shows where to add your highlight, midtone, and contour shades.

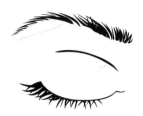
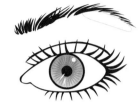
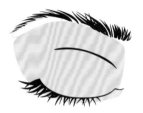
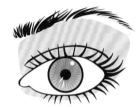
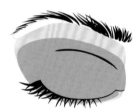
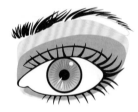

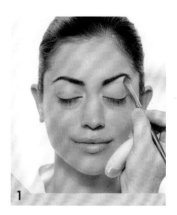

1. With a #22 highlight brush, apply a matte beige eye shadow to just your brow bone—just under the arch of your brow.

2. Curl your eyelashes and apply the first layer of mascara to your top lashes (see page 136).

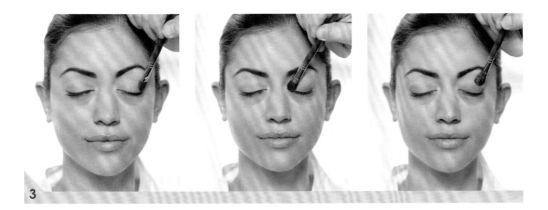

3. With a #27 eye shadow brush (because you will be applying your color to a large area), apply a matte taupe midtone eye shadow. Start at the base of your upper lash line and bring it across the lid, then up and over your entire lid, all the way up to just under your brow bone. By starting along your lash line and working your way upward, you will get the highest concentration of color where you laid your brush first, making your color deeper at the lash line.

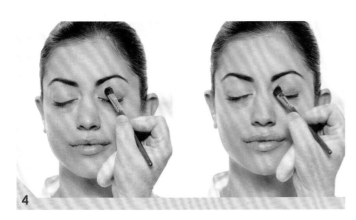

4. With the #27 brush, apply more midtone eye shadow in a half-moon shape all along the crease to create more definition.

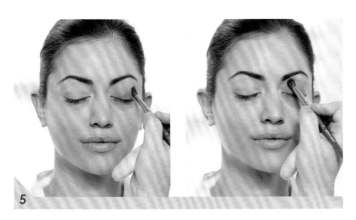

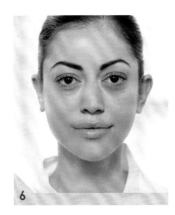

5. Using a #16 blending brush (the one that is always clean and ready to blend with), blend your midtone so there are no hard edges.

6. As you can see, we are starting to acheive a gradation of color with our midtone.

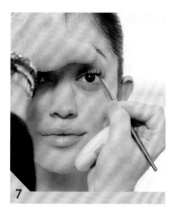

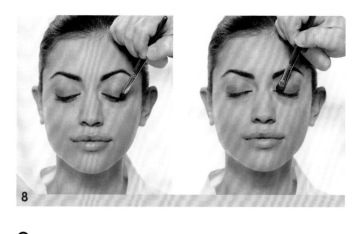

7. To start your lash line definition, use a #41 detail eyeliner brush to push matte black eye shadow into the base of your lash line.

8. With a #30 contour brush and a dark shimmery brown eye shadow, start at the base of your lash line and bring your color up and over your entire lid, up to your crease. This gives you the most intense color right at your lash line.

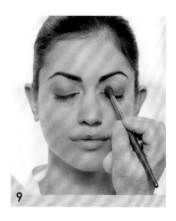

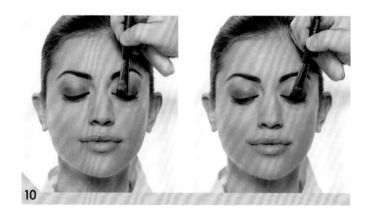

9. Blend with the #16 blending brush.

10. So you don't over-define the eye, apply your false eyelashes now. Start by lining your eyes. To make it softer and look more smudged, use a #18 detail eyeliner brush and lay some matte black shadow all along your top lash line. As you apply it, pull up slightly with your brush to blend the line (see page 130).

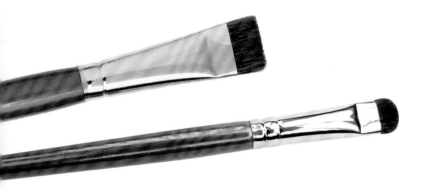

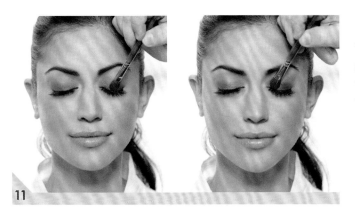

11. After the lash glue has dried, finish the shadow: With a #30 contour brush, apply another layer of dark shimmery brown eye shadow, starting at the base of your lash line and bringing it up over your entire lid, up to your crease, creating more depth at the lash line.

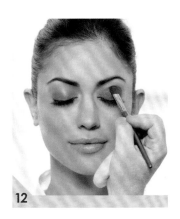

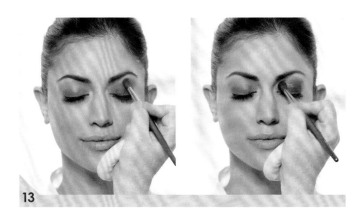

12. Use the #30 contour brush to apply additional dark, shimmery brown eye shadow in a half-moon shape all along your crease and on your lid. Pat it on for more intense color application.

13. Use the #16 blending brush to blend your contour so there are no hard edges.

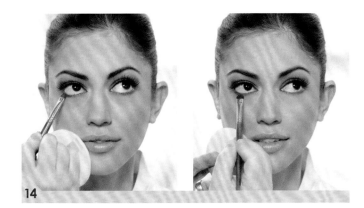

14. With a #38 detail eye shadow brush, apply your midtone shadow all along your lower lash line. Start your application from the outside corner and sweep it across to the inside corner.

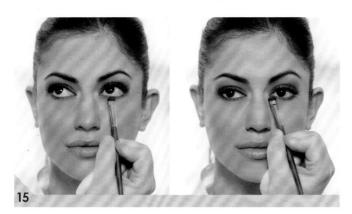

15. With the same brush, apply your contour color right over your midtone all along your lower lash line. By layering on your midtone, then your contour on top of it, you are creating a gradation color, making your lower lash line definition look more natural and blended.

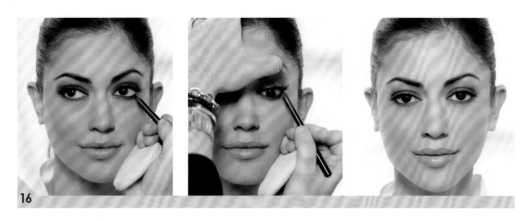

16. Now with a black eyeliner, line the waterline of your lower and upper eyelid. (The waterline is the inner rim of your eye.) This will add just a little more drama to your smoky eye.

17. Finish your eyes with a coat of mascara to the top lashes, blending them into the false eyelashes. Give your bottom lashes a nice coat of mascara.

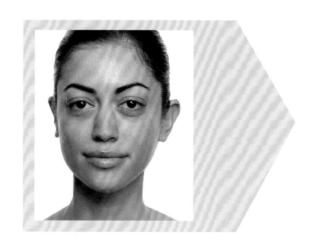

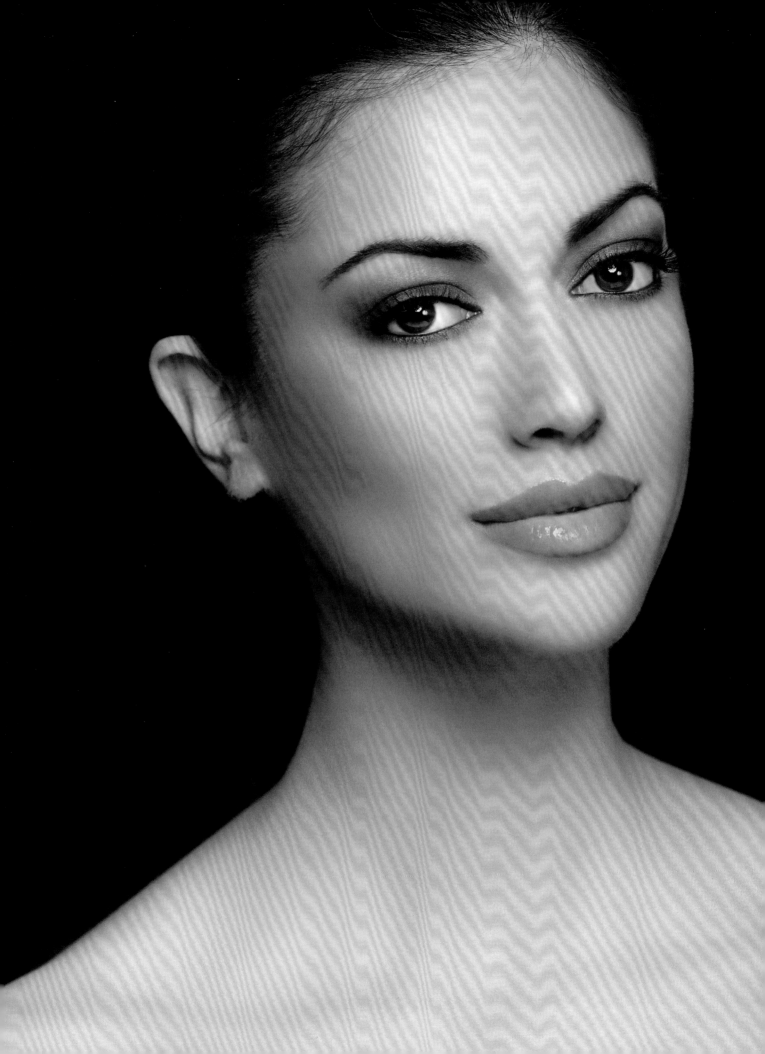

wearable smoky eye

Sometimes you want to wear a more dramatic look but it might not be appropriate. Sometimes you just don't care and do it anyway. But it's nice to have an option for some middle ground. This version of a smoky eye just softens the look slightly, making it easier to wear and more appropriate for those times when a full on smoky eye might be too much.

This diagram shows where to add your highlight, midtone, and contour shades.

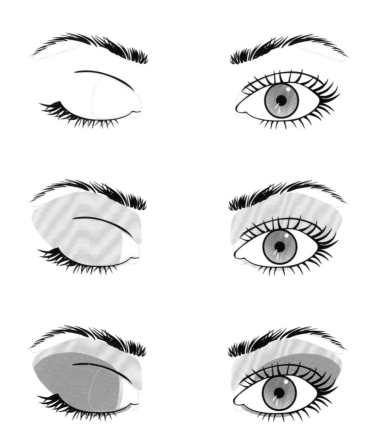

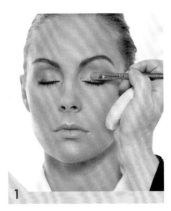

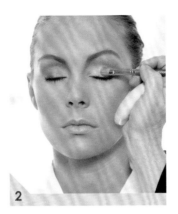

1. Using a #22 highlight brush, apply a crème-to-powder shimmery beige eye shadow to the inside half of your eyelid (just from your lash line to your crease).

2. With the same brush, apply a shimmery champagne powder eye shadow directly on top of the crème.

3. Curl your eyelashes and apply the first layer of mascara to your top lashes (see page 136).

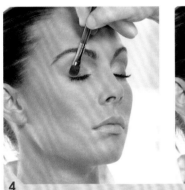

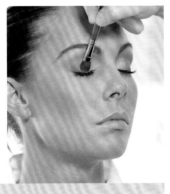

4. With a #27 eye shadow brush (because you're applying color to such a large area), apply a dark matte taupe midtone eye shadow. Start at the base of your upper lash line and bring the color up and over your entire lid. It will overlap the highlight you already put on the lid, muting it. By starting along your lash line and working your way upward, you will get the highest concentration of color where you laid your brush first, making your color depart the lash line.

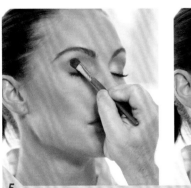

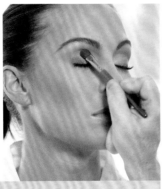

5. With the #27 brush, apply more midtone eye shadow in a half-moon shape all along the crease to create more definition.

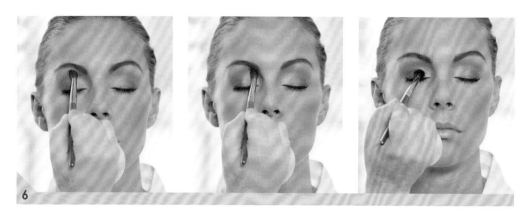

6. Using a #16 blending brush (the one that is always clean and ready to blend with), blend your midtone so there are no hard edges.

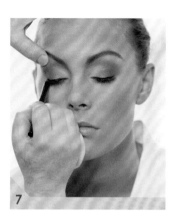

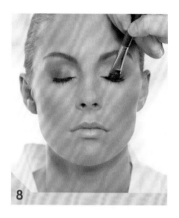

7. To start your lash line definition, use a #41 detail eyeliner brush to push matte black shadow into the base of your lash line. Follow it by using a black eyeliner to line all along your top lash line.

8. Soften the line using a #18 detail eyeliner brush and a matte black eye shadow by going over the line and smudging it.

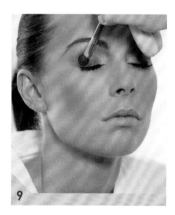

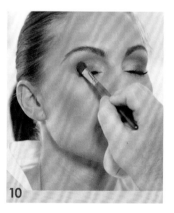

9. With a #27 eye shadow brush and a dark shimmery golden brown eye shadow, start at the base of your lash line, work it across the lid, and bring it up and over the entire lid, up to your crease. This gives you the most intense color right at your lash line. It too will also slightly overlap the highlight shade you applied earlier.

10. Use the #27 brush to apply additional dark, shimmery golden brown eye shadow in a half-moon shape all along your crease and on your lid. Pat it on for more intense color application.

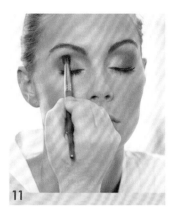

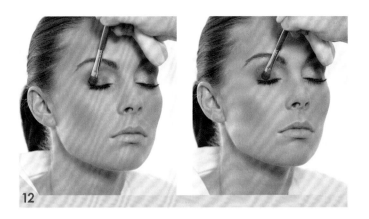

11. Use the #16 blending brush and blend your contour so there are no hard edges.

12. With a #30 contour brush, apply another layer of dark shimmery golden brown eye shadow all along the upper lash line for more intense color.

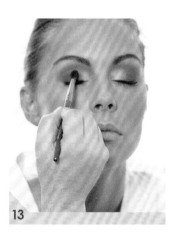

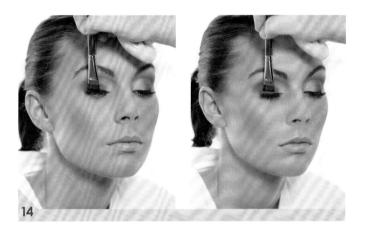

13. Follow with the #16 blending brush to blend.

14. To create more intensity at the lash line, use the #18 eyeliner brush to grab some matte black shadow and lay your brush at your lash line. Pull up slightly to blend out and smudge the color. Do this all the way across your upper lash line.

15. For a little more drama, apply false eyelashes (see page 188).

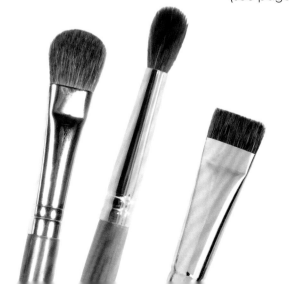

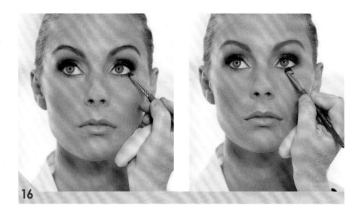

16. With a #38 detail eye shadow brush, apply your midtone shadow all along your lower lash line. Once again, start your application from the outside corner, sweeping it across to the inside corner.

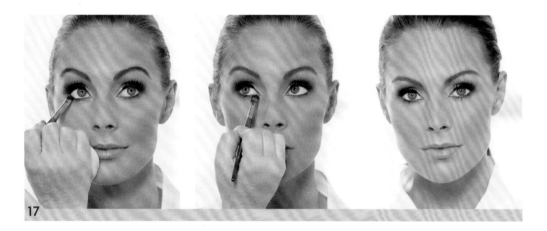

17. With the same brush, apply your contour color over your midtone all along your lower lash line. By layering on your midtone, then your contour on top of it, you are creating a gradation of color, making your lower lash line definition look more natural and blended.

18. Finish your eyes by applying a coat of mascara to the top lashes, blending them into the false eyelashes. Last, give your bottom lashes a coat of mascara.

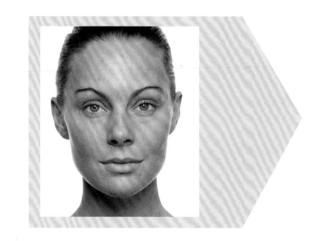

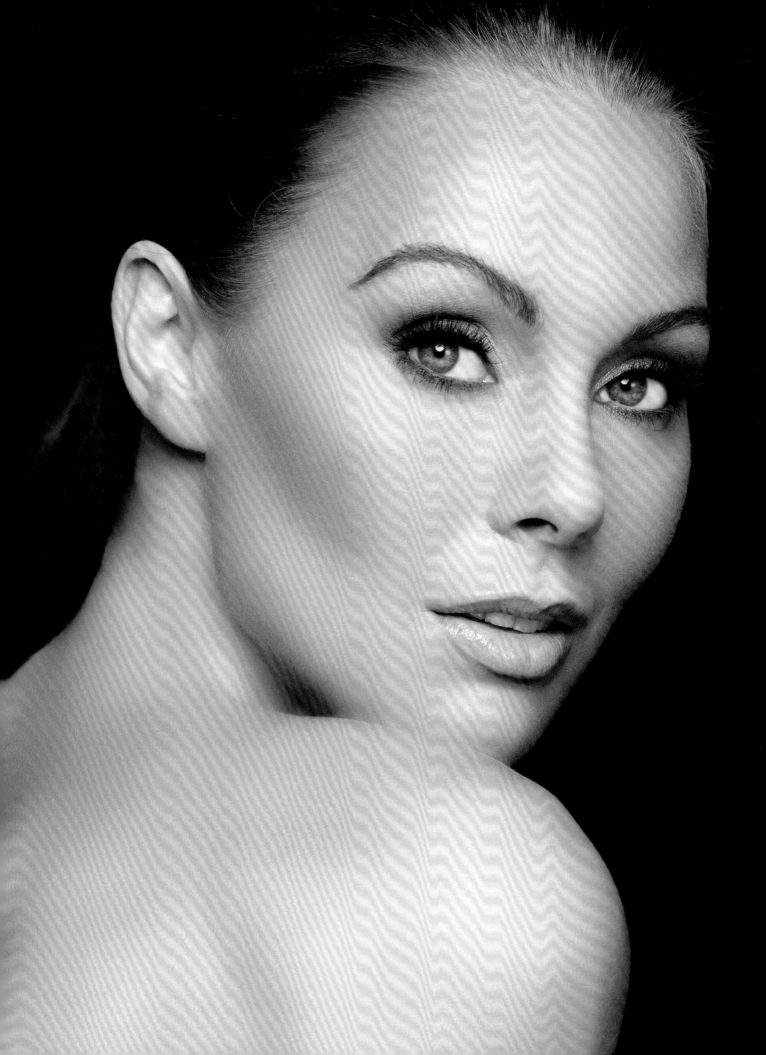

modern audrey eye

This is a classic, named after one of the most iconic beauties of all times because it was her signature look. This is my modern take on Audrey Hepburn's classic look—a look that's easy to wear but not necessarily easy to do. I'm going to show you a trick that makes it easier to achieve.

This diagram shows where to add your highlight, midtone, and contour shades.

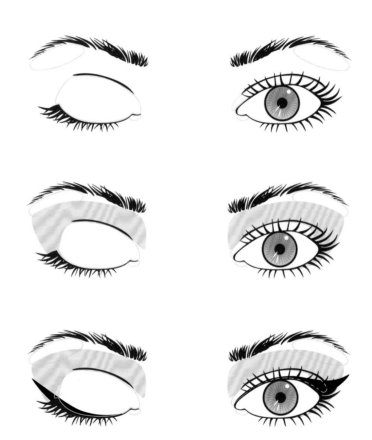

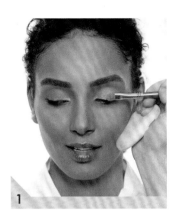

1. Using your #22 highlight brush, apply a crème-to-powder shimmery gold eye shadow to your eyelid (just from your lash line to your crease).

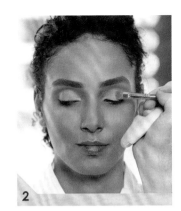

2. With the same brush, apply a shimmery gold eye shadow directly on top of the crème to create a beautiful sheen.

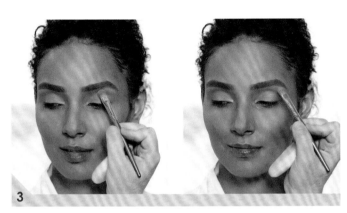

3. Again with the same brush, apply a matte flesh eye shadow to your brow bone—the area just under the arch of your brow.

4. Curl your eyelashes and apply the first layer of mascara to your top lashes (see page 136).

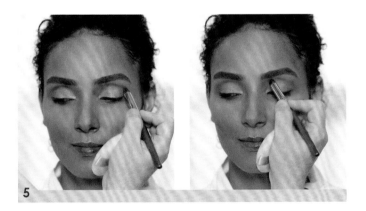

5. With this look, you want your midtone very precise so it defines the shape without darkening your lid. Because this look has such an intense and dramatic liner, you want your lid soft and shimmery. Using your #20 ultimate crease brush, apply your matte ginger midtone eye shadow in your crease. Starting from the outside corner of your crease, glide your brush across to the inside corner, creating a distinct line all along your crease.

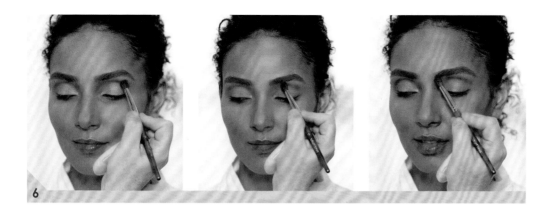

6. Using your #16 blending brush (the one that is always clean and ready to blend with), blend out your midtone so there are no hard edges. Just retrace the same area you just applied your midtone to, rather than blending it up and down to darken too much of your lid.

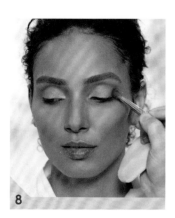

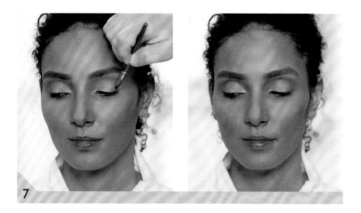

7. With your #38 detail eye shadow brush, apply midtone just to the outer edge of your lid.

8. Blend with your #16 blending brush, making sure to keep the color to the very outer edge of your lid.

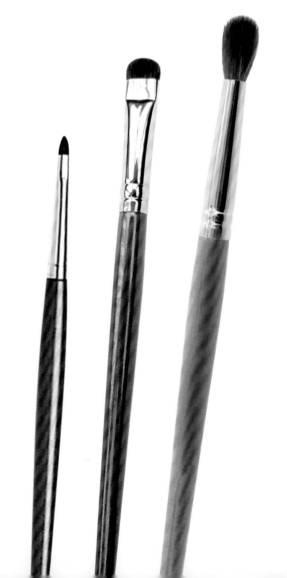

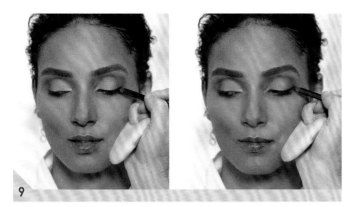

9. Create that perfect dramatic liner along your top lid: The trick is layering it in steps. Even pros prefer to layer. First, begin to create a pattern with a black eyeliner pencil because it is easier to remove and start over if you make a mistake. Starting at the inside corner of your top lash line, slowly move across the lash line. Make sure your line is its most narrow at the inside corner, gradually getting thicker as you reach the outside corner. As you reach the outside corner, you can give it a little kick upward.

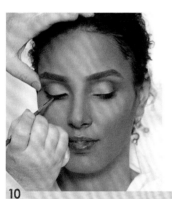
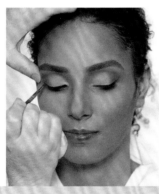

10. Your penciling probably won't be perfect, but it doesn't have to be because you are now going to trace over it with a matte black eye shadow and your #42 eyeliner brush to perfect your pattern.

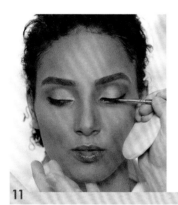
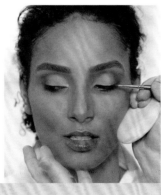
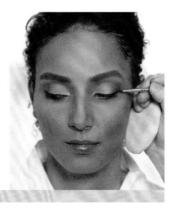

11. I know your line looks perfect now, but it's still not dramatic enough! Go over your pattern with your liquid or gel eyeliner. Because you created the pattern, even if your liquid isn't perfect, it won't show. Using your #42 eyeliner brush, apply your liquid or gel, starting from the inside corner and working toward the outer corner. Follow your pattern.

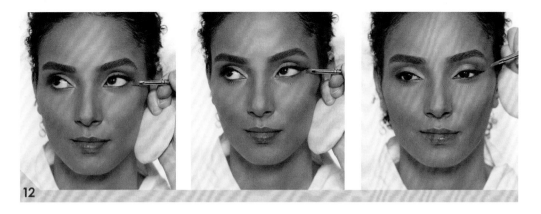

12. Any mistakes can be fixed with a little concealer and your #50 concealer brush.

13. For the perfect amount of drama, apply false eyelashes (see page 188).

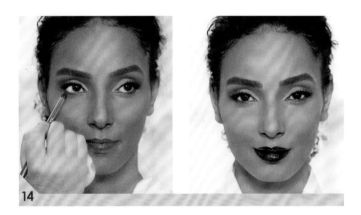

14. Using your #13 detail eye shadow brush, apply your midtone eye shadow along the outside corner of the lower lash line to close in the outer corner of the eye.

15. Finish the eye by applying a layer of mascara to your top lashes, blending them into the false eyelashes.

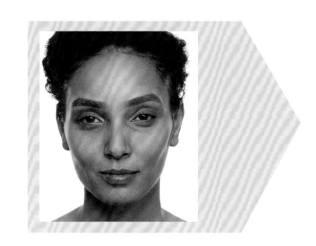

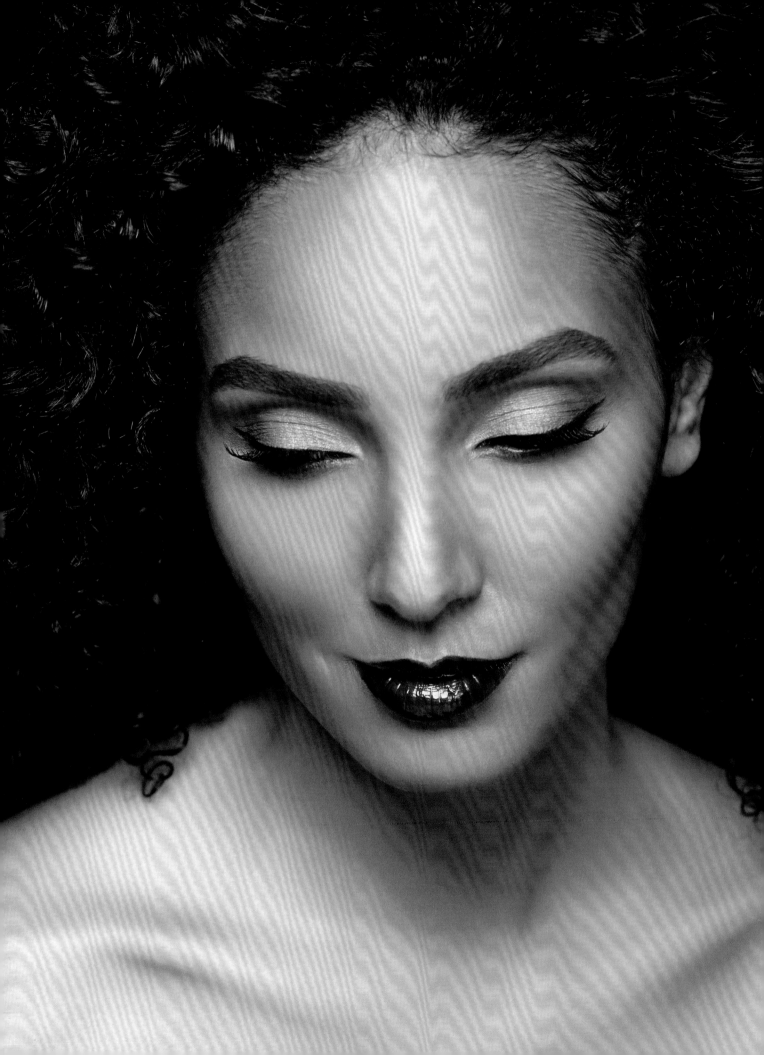

sparkling eye

This is one of my favorite looks. It works wonderfully for photos and special occasions. It's all about creating the most shape possible with the eyelid, which is why it photographs so beautifully. Contrast is not only created with color, but with texture.

One of the most important aspects of contrast in this look is shimmer versus matte. By using shimmer against matte, you create an even greater contrast, which increases the visual illusion you are creating with your shadows. The pieces you are visually pushing forward and pulling back appear to be more dramatically placed.

It's imperative that the only place you use any shimmer or frost is on the eyelid (your highlight shade), so it increases the appearance of its effect. Your midtone and contour are absolutely matte. Also, your highlight should be quite light in depth, with your contour quite deep. Between the texture and the color depth difference, it completely increases the shaping of the lid, which looks amazing. It also allows you to create all kinds of effects, such as a fake crease, which is why I love using this technique so much.

This diagram shows where to add your highlight, midtone, and contour shades.

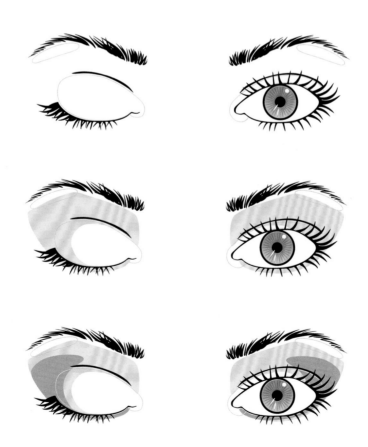

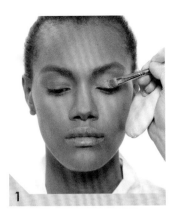

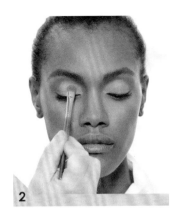

1. Using your #22 highlight brush, apply a crème-to-powder shimmery gold eye shadow to your lid (just from the lash line to your crease). You are going to layer crème and powder to make your lid more dramatic.

2. With the same brush, apply a shimmery peachy gold eye shadow directly on top of the crème. Pat it on to get more color application.

3. Curl your eyelashes and apply the first layer of mascara to your top lashes (see page 136).

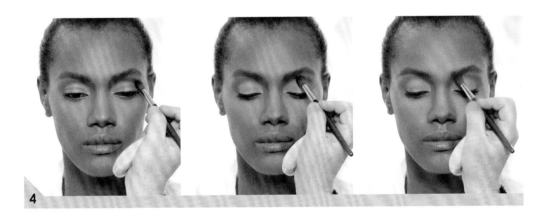

4. Using your #11 midtone brush and a matte midtone, starting from the outside corner of your crease, glide your brush across to the inside corner. Use a matte ginger eye shadow (a shade just a bit darker than your skin tone) so you get soft definition.

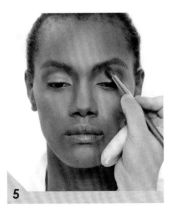

5. Using your #16 blending brush (the one that is always clean and ready to blend with), blend out your midtone so there are no hard edges.

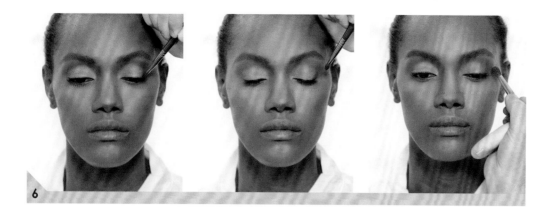

6. With your #30 contour brush and some midtone, define the outer corner of your eyelid. Follow with your #16 blending brush to blend.

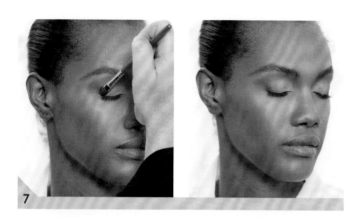

7. With your #30 contour brush, apply a dark matte brown eye shadow on the outer corner of your eyelid and up into the crease. You are layering it over your midtone so it starts to create a blend.

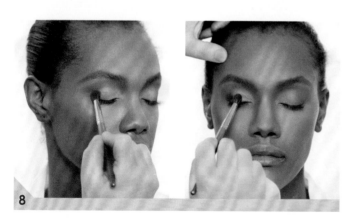

8. Follow with your #16 blending brush to blend out your contour color up toward your crease and in toward your lid.

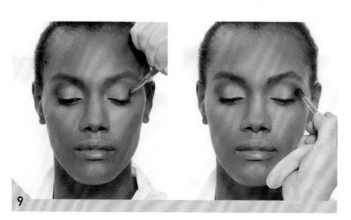

9. With your #30 contour brush, apply another layer of your contour color, building up to create depth, followed with your #16 blending brush to blend out.

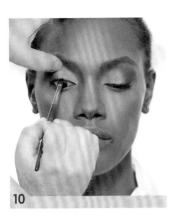

10. To start your lash line definition, use your #41 detail eyeliner brush to push matte black eye shadow into the base of your lash line. Follow it by using a black eyeliner to line all along your top lash line.

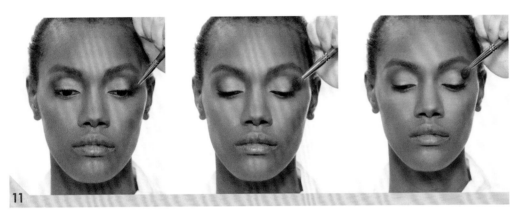

11. With your #30 contour brush, apply another layer of your contour color, building it up to create depth, followed with your #16 blending brush to blend out.

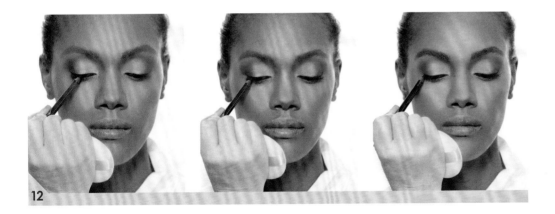

12. To create more definition at the lash line, line your eyes with black eyeliner right along the lash line, keeping the line as close to the lash line as possible. Make sure it is the thinnest at the inside corner, slowly getting thicker as you get to the outside corner.

13. For the perfect amount of drama, apply false eyelashes (see page 188).

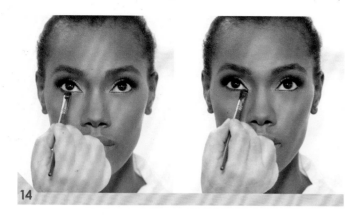

14. With your #38 detail eye shadow brush, apply your mid-tone all along your lower lash line. Start your application from the outside corner, sweeping it across to the inside corner.

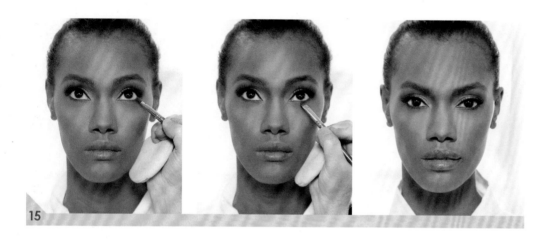

15. With the same brush, apply a layer of your contour color right over your midtone all along your bottom lash line. By layering your midtone on, then applying your contour on top of it, you are creating a gradation of color, making your lower lash line definition look more natural and blended.

16. Using your #14 detail highlight brush, highlight the inside corner of the lower lash line. This really brightens the eye and opens it up to give you a wide-eyed effect.

17. Finish the eyes by applying a coat of mascara to the top lashes, blending them into your false eyelashes. Lastly, give your bottom lashes a nice coat of mascara.

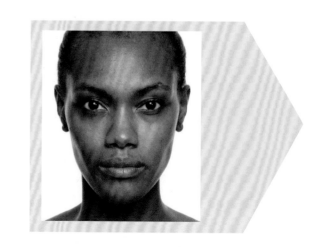

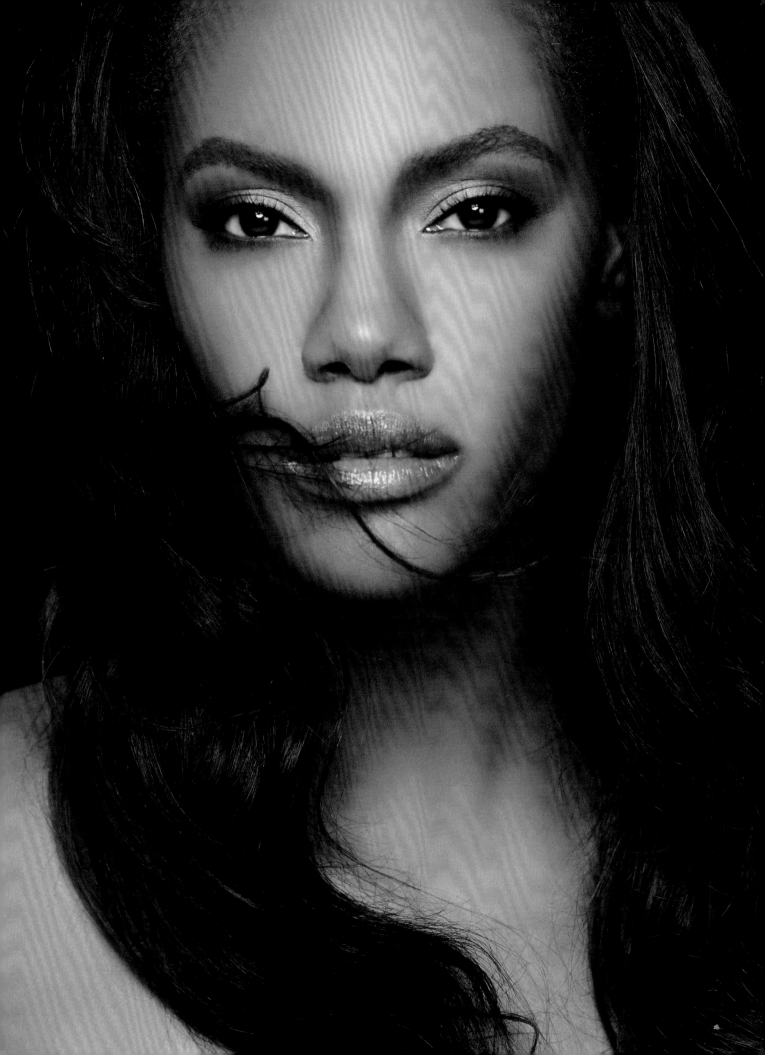

playing with color

There is a trick to using bright color well. Bright colors cannot reshape the eyelid, so you need to do all your shaping first with neutrals. Then layer your bright colors on top. And yes, the brights will still be vivid!

You can first paint and shape your eyes with neutral shades to help bring them out. Then layer your bright colors right on top of your neutrals. That way you get great shape to the lid while still getting a great shot of fun bright color.

This diagram shows where to add your highlight, midtone, and contour shades.

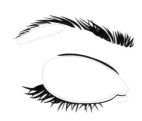
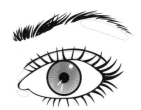

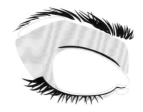
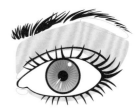

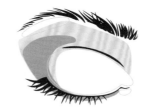
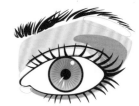

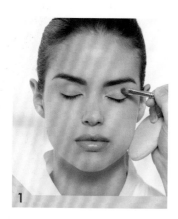

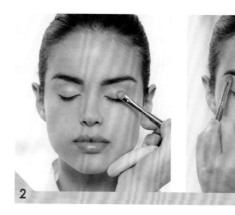

1. Using your #22 highlight brush, apply a crème-to-powder shimmery beige eye shadow to your lid (from your lash line to your crease). You are going to layer crème and powder to make your lid more dramatic.

2. With the same brush, apply a shimmery champagne eye shadow directly on top of the crème and also apply it to your brow bone—right under your arch.

3. Curl your eyelashes and apply the first layer of mascara to your top lashes (see page 136).

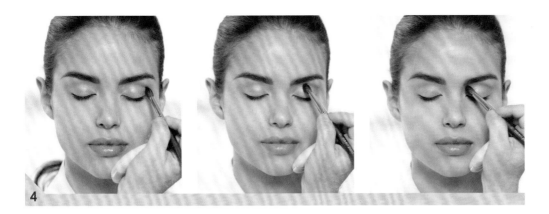

4. Using your #11 midtone brush and a matte midtone eye shadow, start from the outside corner of your eye and glide your brush across to the inside corner. Use a soft matte caramel shadow (a shade just a bit darker than your skin tone) to get soft definition.

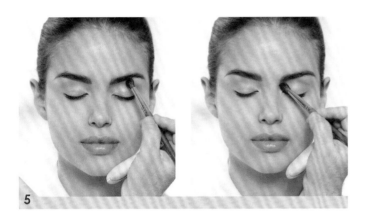

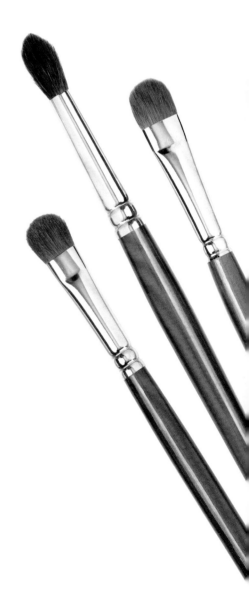

5. Using your #16 blending brush (the one that is always clean and ready to blend with), blend your midtone so there are no hard edges.

6. Add another layer for more definition.

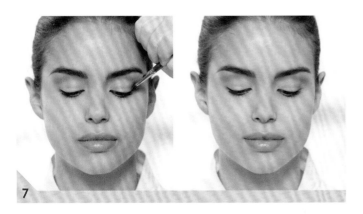

7. Use your #30 contour brush and some midtone shadow to define the outer corner of your eyelid.

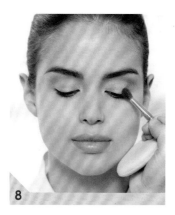

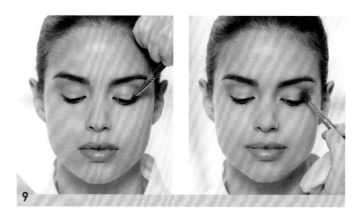

8. Follow with your #16 blending brush and blend toward the inside. This gives you just a hint of definition and color.

9. Add another layer for more definition and to help support the bright color you're about to apply.

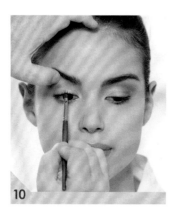

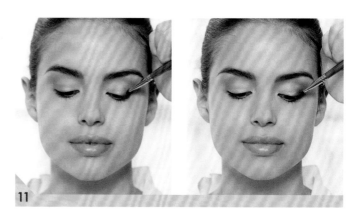

10. To start your lash line definition, use your #41 detail eyeliner brush to push matte black eye shadow into the base of your lash line. Follow it by using a black eyeliner to line all along your top lash line.

11. Create lid shape before adding your bright color. With your #30 contour brush, apply a shimmery pinky gray eye shadow on the outer corner of your eyelid. You are layering it over your midtone so it starts to create a blend.

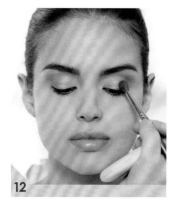

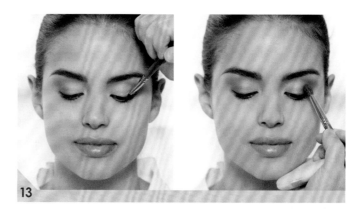

12. With your #16 blending brush, blend your color up toward your crease and in toward your lid.

13. Add another layer for more depth to support the bright color you're about to add.

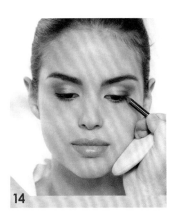

14. To create more definition at the lash line, line your eyes with a black eyeliner right along the lash line, keeping the line as close to the lash line as possible. Make sure it is the thinnest at the inside corner, slowly getting thicker as you get to the outside corner.

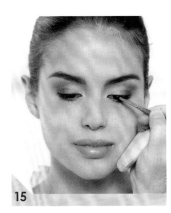

15. Smooth your liner with your #42 eyeliner brush so it is slightly smudged and blended.

16. For the perfect amount of drama, apply false eyelashes (see page 188).

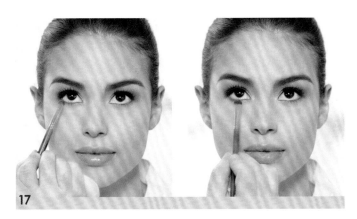

17. With your #38 detail eye shadow brush, apply your midtone all along your lower lash line. Start your application from the outside corner, sweeping it across to the inside corner.

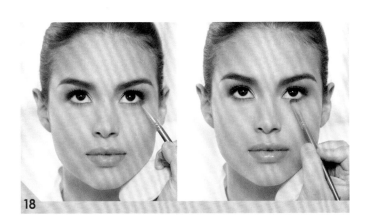

18. With the same brush, apply a layer of shimmery pinky gray color right over your midtone all along your bottom lash line. By layering your midtone on, then applying your contour on top of it, you are creating a gradation of color, making your lower lash line definition look more natural and blended and creating shape before you apply your bright color.

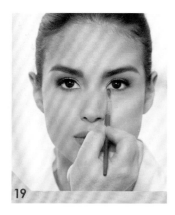

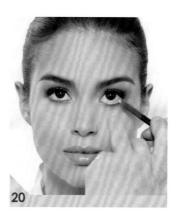

19. Using your #14 detail highlight brush, highlight the inside corner of the lower lash line with shimmery champagne eye shadow. This really brightens the eye and opens it up to give you a wide-eyed effect.

20. To make your eyes look even bigger when finished, line your waterline with a beige concealer pencil. (The waterline is the inner rim of your eye.)

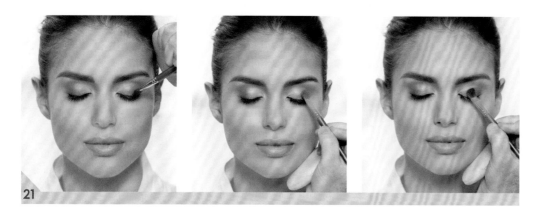

21. Add a sheer wash of an iridescent purple. Using your #30 contour brush, apply a sheer shimmery iridescent purple to the outer third of the eyelid. Pat it on for more concentrated application of color.

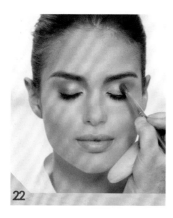

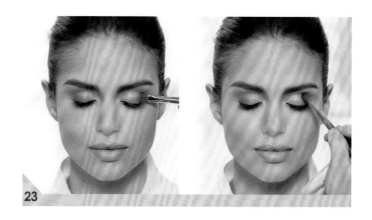

22. Using your #16 blending brush, blend your color up into your crease and over your lid, toward the inside corner, about halfway.

23. Apply another layer for depth and a pop of color.

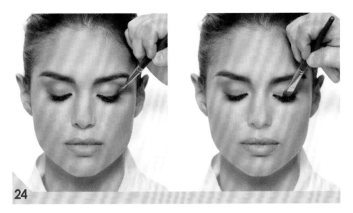

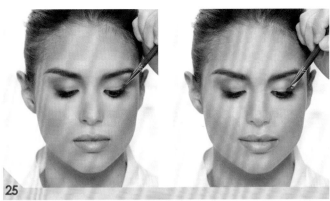

24. With your #22 highlight brush, apply a dark purple crème shadow at the base of the lash line in the outer corner of the lid to help create color and depth. (When you layer crème and powder, it will intensify the color.)

25. Using your #38 detail eye shadow brush you can get your eye shadow right at the lash line, apply your bright rich dark purple shadow right on top of your crème purple shadow. Be sure and pat on plenty of color so you have plenty to blend up and out.

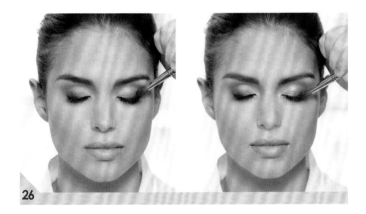

26. With your #16 blending brush, blend your bright rich dark purple eye shadow up toward your crease and onto the outer third of your lid.

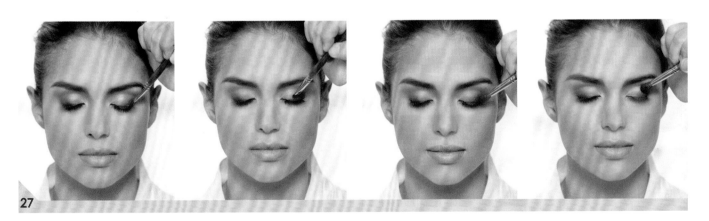

27. Keep layering on more purple until you get the intensity you are looking for. Pat the eye shadow on close to the lash line for intense color application and then blend up and out.

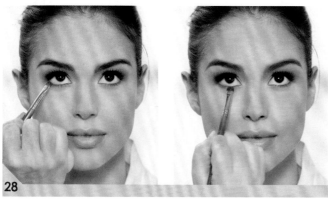

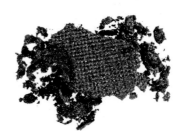

28. Using your #38 detail eye shadow brush, layer purple eye shadow all along your lower lash line right on top of the color you applied earlier.

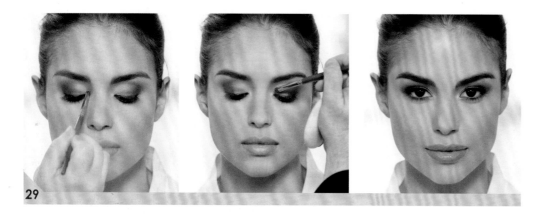

29. To increase contrast, add another layer of shimmery champagne eye shadow to the inner corner of your eyelid top and bottom with your #14 detail highlight brush. It will make the purple look more intense.

30. Finish with a layer of mascara on your bottom lashes and another layer on top, blending them into your false eyelashes.

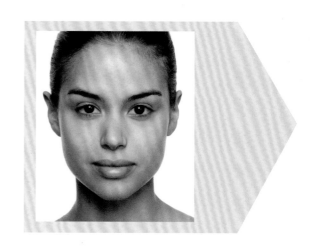

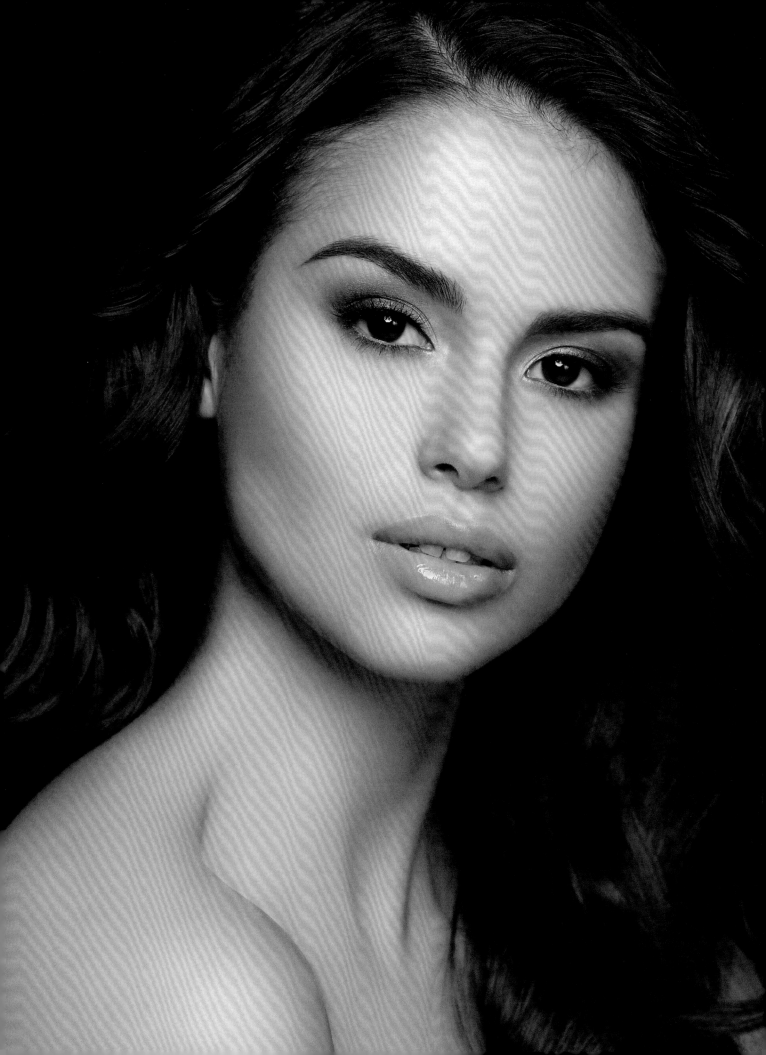

brigitte bardot

Another iconic woman with an iconic look—known for her sultriness, Brigitte Bardot was not credited with creating the smoky eye, but with making it an everyday look. Hers was, of course, her own modern take on the classic look. Now here's my modern take on her classic look.

What makes this smoky eye different is that it is always matte, and the smoke is always kept closer to the lash line and less blended up toward the crease. The matte-ness and the tightness of the color is what makes it more wearable at all times. You don't want to use black because your goal is for it to be softer, but still completely sexy.

This diagram shows where to add your highlight, midtone, and contour shades.

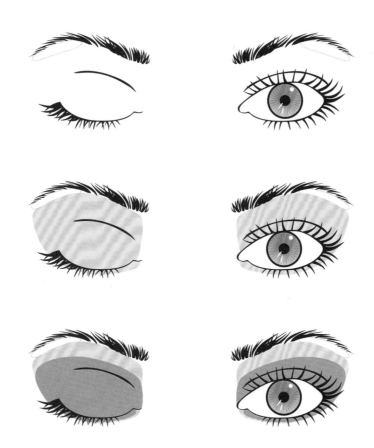

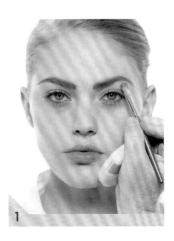

1. With a #22 highlight brush, apply a matte beige eye shadow just to your brow bone—the arch of your brow.

2. Curl your eyelashes and apply the first layer of mascara to your top lashes (see page 136).

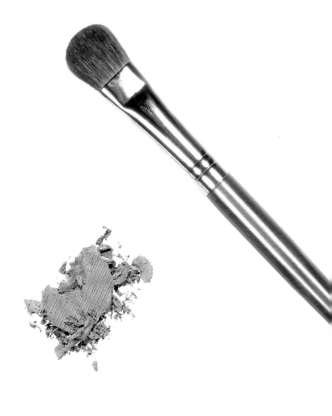

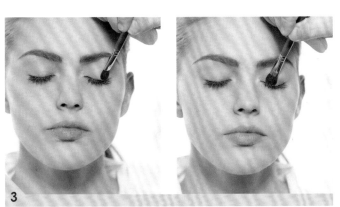

3. With a #27 eye shadow brush (because you will be applying your color to a large area), apply a matte taupe midtone eye shadow. Start at the base of your upper lash line, bring it across the lid, and then bring the color up and over your entire lid, all the way up to just under your brow bone. By starting along your lash line and working your way upward, you will get the highest concentration of color where you laid your brush first, making your color deepest at the lash line.

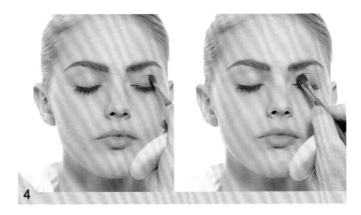

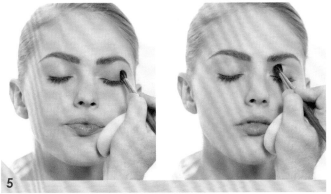

4. With the #27 brush, apply more midtone eye shadow in a half-moon shape all along the crease to create more definition.

5. Using a #16 blending brush (the one that is always clean and ready to blend with), blend your midtone so there are no hard edges.

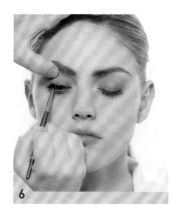

6. To start your lash line definition, use a #41 eyeliner brush to push matte black eye shadow into the base of your lash line.

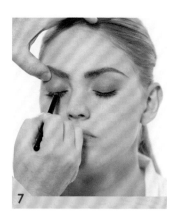

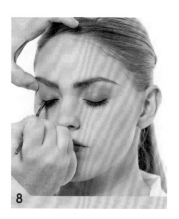

7. To create more definition at the lash line, line your eyes with a black eyeliner right along the lash line, keeping the line as close to the lash line as possible. Make sure it is the thinnest at the inside corner, slowly getting thicker as you get to the outside corner.

8. Smooth your liner with a #42 eyeliner brush to make sure it is slightly smudged and blended.

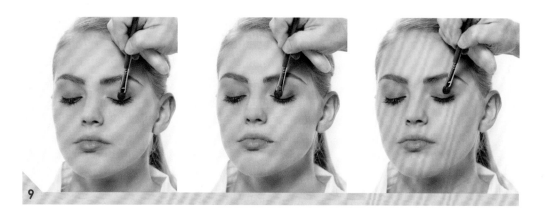

9. With a #30 contour shadow brush, use a matte brown eye shadow, starting at the base of your lash line, and bring your color up and over your entire lid up toward your crease. This gives you the most intense color right at your lash line.

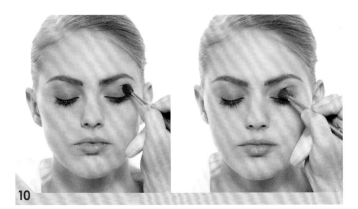

10. Blend the line with the #16 blending brush.

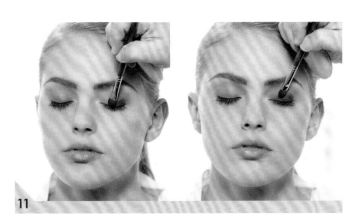

11. With the #30 contour shadow brush, apply another layer of matte brown eye shadow, keeping it close to the lash line when you apply it.

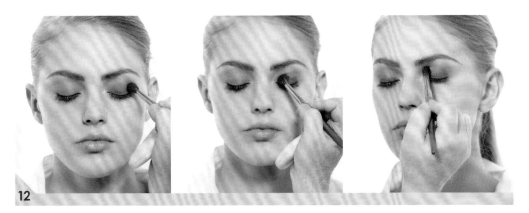

12. With the #16 blending brush, start to blend, keeping your blend tight to the lash line at first and then slowly starting to blend up toward your crease. Keep the most intense color more toward the lash line.

13. For the perfect amount of drama, apply false eyelashes (see page 188).

14. To make your eyeliner softer and more smudged, use a #18 eyeliner brush to grab some matte black eye shadow and lay it all along your top lash line. As you apply it, pull up slightly with your brush to blend the line (see page 130).

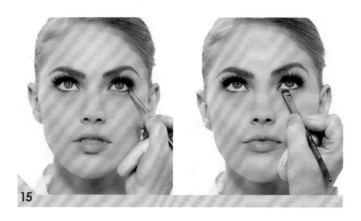

15. With the #38 detail eye shadow brush, apply your midtone eye shadow all along your lower lash line. Once again, start your application from the outside corner, sweeping it across to the inside corner.

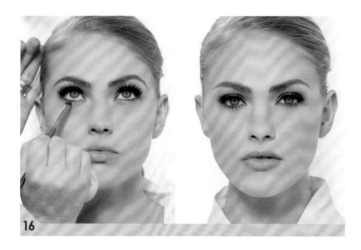

16. With the same brush, apply your contour color right over your midtone all along your lower lash line. By layering on your midtone, then your contour on top of it, you are creating a gradation of color, making your lower lash line definition look more natural and blended.

17. Finish with a layer of mascara on your bottom lashes and another layer on your top, blending them into your false eyelashes.

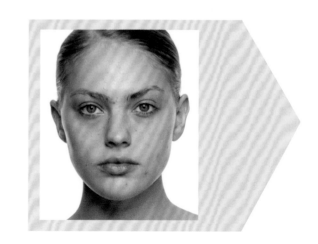

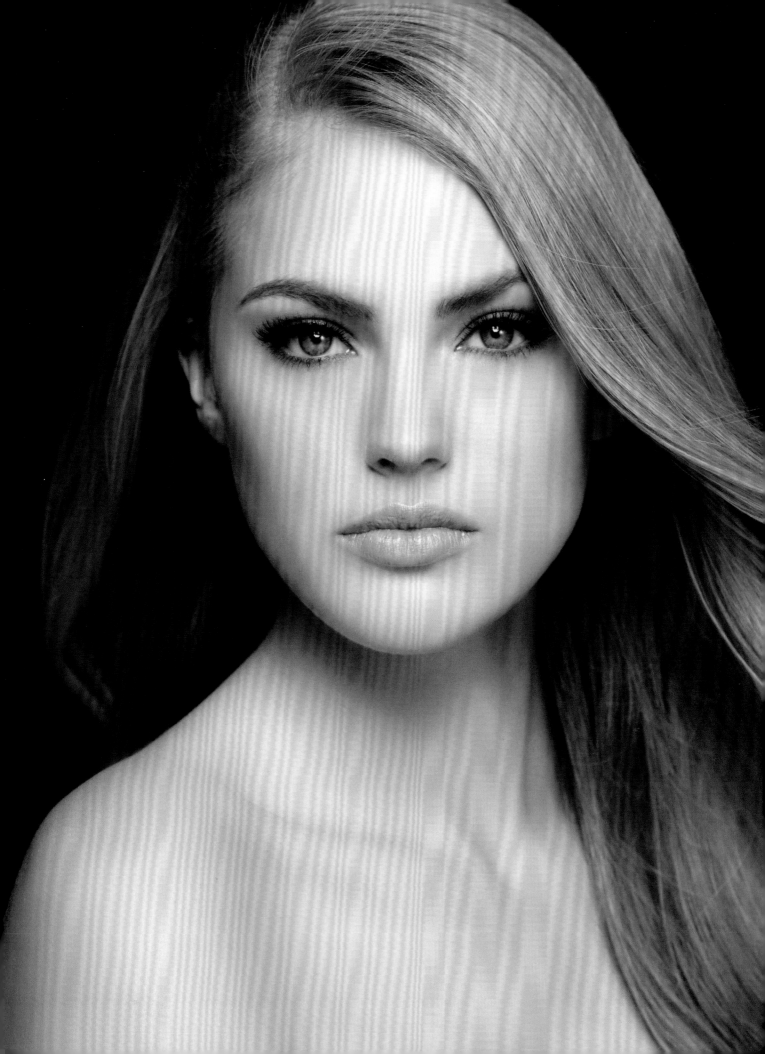

marilyn

Yet another icon—you only need her first name to know who she is. Her name is synonymous with glamour. She was known for her undeniable sexiness and beauty. Her look was all about understated glamour. All about a shimmery lid with a defined crease.

Again, this is my modern take on a classic look, but the theory of the application is still the same. It is all about creating a fake crease; you choose where and how intense the crease is. It's a shimmery lid with a deepened controlled crease and lots of definition at the lash line.

This diagram shows where to add your highlight, midtone, and contour shades.

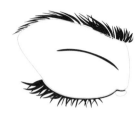
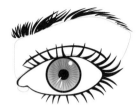
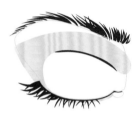
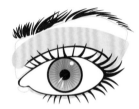
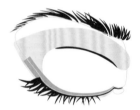
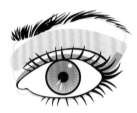

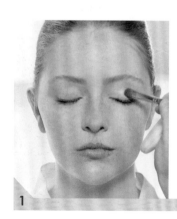
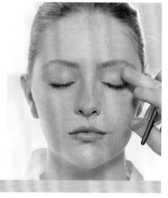

1. Using your #22 highlight brush, apply a crème-to-powder shimmery beige eye shadow, but only to your lid (from the lash line to your crease). You are going to layer crème and powder to make your lid more dramatic.

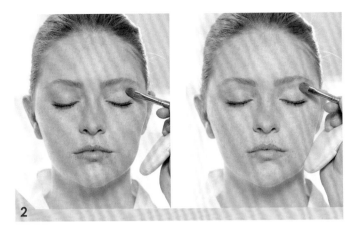

2. With the same brush, apply a shimmery champagne eye shadow and a matte beige directly on top of the crème. Combining a matte and a shimmer will give you more complete coverage, creating a more dramatic lid. Take this eye shadow up to your brow bone so you have a canvas on which to create your crease.

3. Curl your eyelashes and apply the first layer of mascara to your top lashes (see page 136).

4. To start your lash line definition, use your #41 detail eyeliner brush to push matte black eye shadow into the base of your lash line.

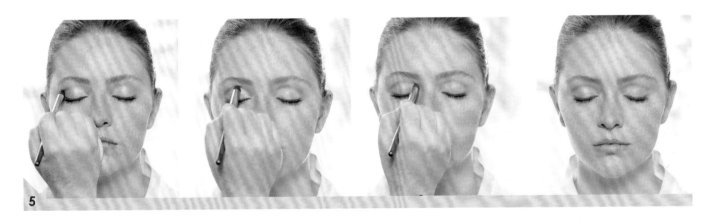

5. With this look, you want your midtone very precise, so it won't darken your lid but define the shape. You want your lids shimmery and defined. Using your #20 ultimate crease eye shadow brush, apply your matte taupe midtone shadow in your crease: Starting from the outside corner of your crease, glide your brush across to the inside corner. Create a distinct line all along your crease. You may even want to apply a couple of layers so it is very defined.

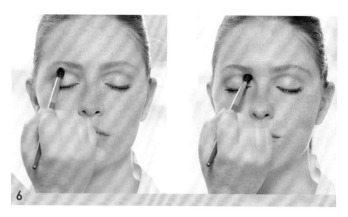 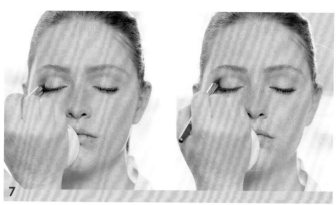

6. Using your #16 blending brush (the one that is always clean and ready to blend with), blend out your midtone so there are no hard edges. But make sure you just retrace the same area that you applied your midtone in the previous step. Don't blend it up and down or you'll darken too much of your lid.

7. Now, for a little extra definition. Using your #20 eye shadow brush, add some of your midtone eye shadow, but just to the very outermost corner of your eyelid, right along your lash line and up into the outer part of your crease, much like the letter v. This will close in the eyelid and help start your lid definition.

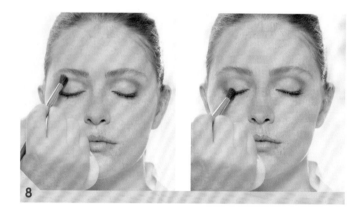

8. Blend with your #16 blending brush, keeping your blend very tight.

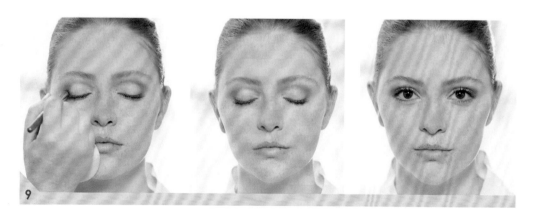

9. Keep layering until you get the depth that you desire.

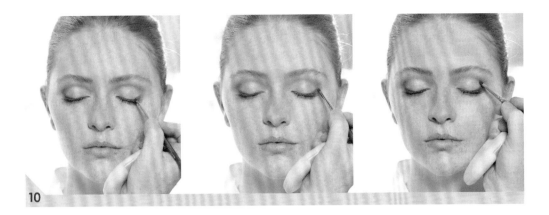

10. Now, start your lash line definition: Use your #42 eye liner brush and a matte brown eye shadow to apply shadow right along the lash line, bringing it up into the outer edge of your crease for nice subtle definition.

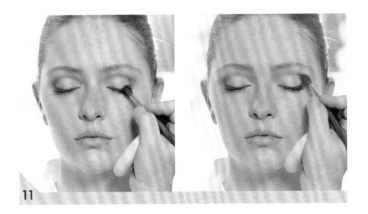

11. Using your #16 blending brush, blend the color out, being very careful to keep the color nice and tight.

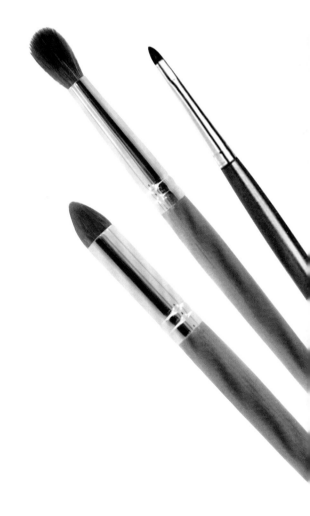

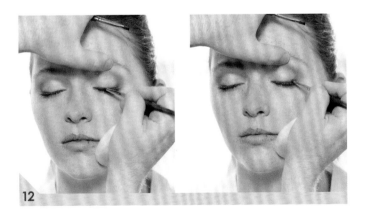

12. Apply another layer all along your lash line for more definition.

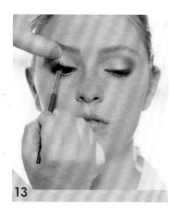

13. For even more definition, use your #41 detail eyeliner brush to push matte black eye shadow into the base of your lash line. This will make your eyelashes look thicker and start to define your lash line.

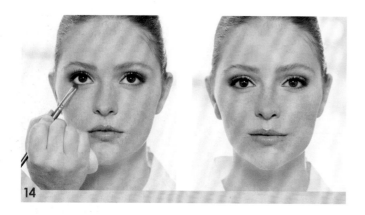

14. With your #38 detail eye shadow brush, apply your midtone all along your lower lash line. Start from the outside corner and work in toward the inner corner.

15. Using your #14 detail highlight brush, highlight the inside corner of your lower lash line.

16. Finish with another layer of mascara on your top lashes.

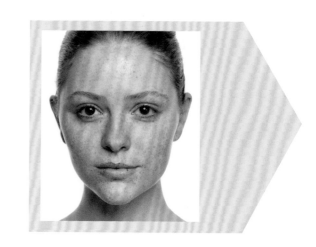

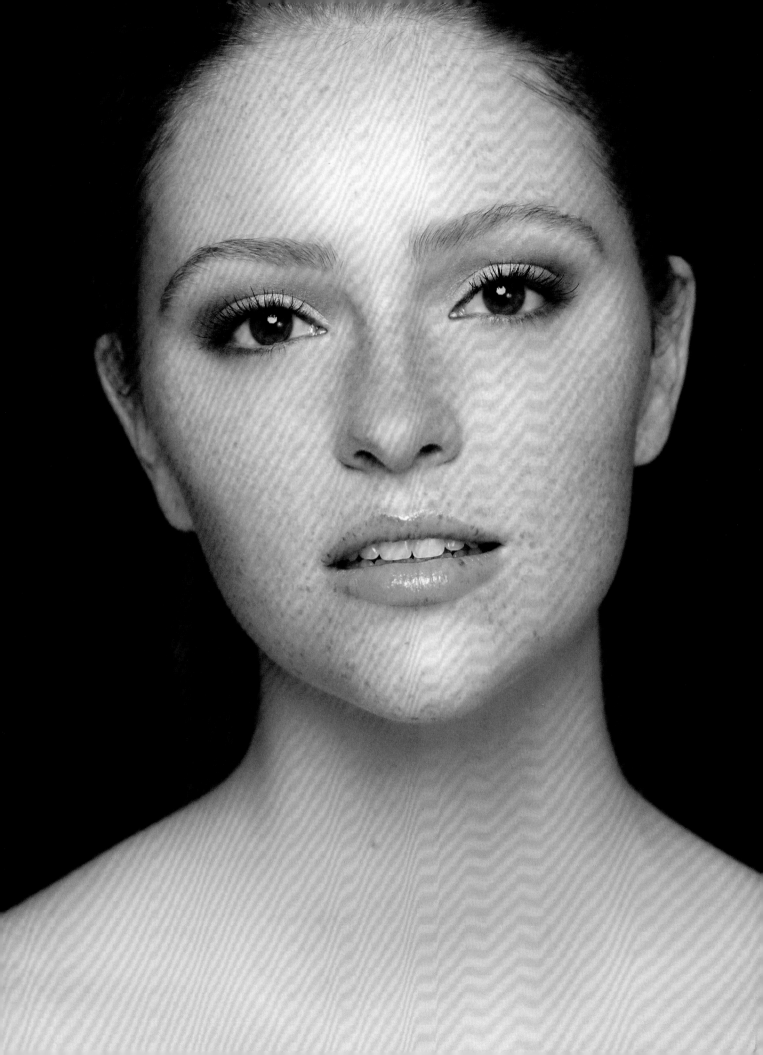

smoking
with crèmes

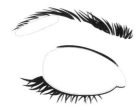
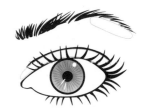

Some would call this a very rock 'n' roll look, because of the smudginess of the smoky eye. I just like the kind of slept-in look it has. The great part of creating a smoky eye with a crème is that it is fast. The hard part is blending, but you will conquer it with a little practice.

This diagram shows where to add your highlight, midtone, and contour shades.

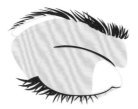
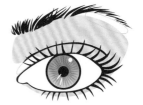

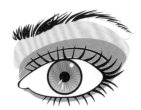

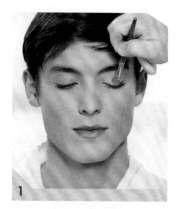

1. With a #22 highlight brush, apply a shimmery champagne eye shadow all along your lid up to your crease.

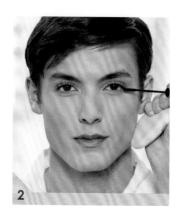

2. Curl your eyelashes and apply the first layer of mascara to your top lashes (see page 136).

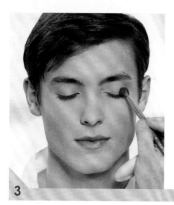
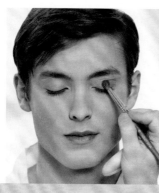

3. Using a #16 blending brush so your color will be soft and blended as you apply it, apply a matte mid-tone eye shadow starting from the outside corner of your eye, gliding your brush across to the inside corner. Also apply it to the outer half of the eyelid. Use a soft matte taupe eye shadow (a shade just a bit darker than your skin tone) to get soft definition.

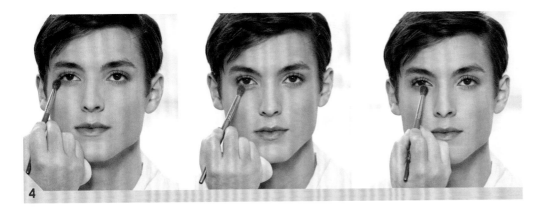

4. With the same brush, apply your midtone all along your lower lash line.

5. This will create very smudged out color because of the size and shape of the brush you are using.

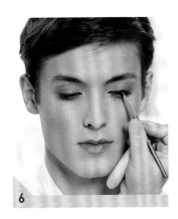

6. To start your lash line definition, use a #41 detail eyeliner brush to push matte black eye shadow into the base of your lash line.

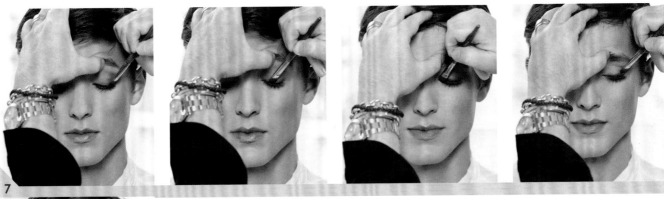

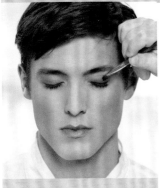

7. With a fresh #22 highlight brush and a matte black crème eye shadow, start at the base of your lash line and bring your color up and over your entire lid up toward your crease. This gives you the most intense color right at your lash line.

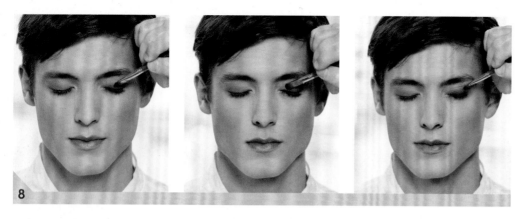

8. Keep layering it until you get the intensity you desire, always stating at the lash line.

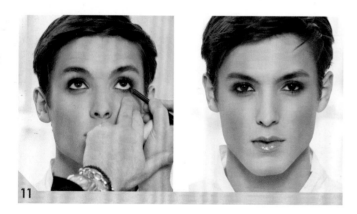

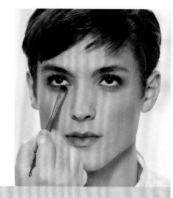

9. Use a clean #30 contour brush to blend where your crème shadow blends into your crease. You are using a #30 contour brush instead of a normal blending brush because the bristles are stiffer, which is better for blending a crème shadow.

10. With the #22 highlight brush, apply some of your black crème eye shadow all along your lower lash line, smudging it out and dragging it down a little as you go across to create that smudginess.

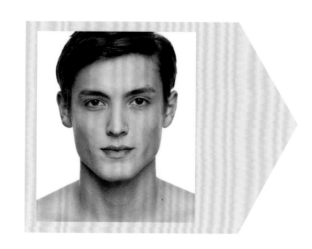

11. With a black eyeliner, line the waterline of your lower and upper eyelids. (The waterline is the inner rim of your eye.) This will add just a little more drama to your smoky eye.

12. Finish your eyes by applying a coat of mascara to the top lashes. Lastly, give your bottom lashes a nice coat of mascara.

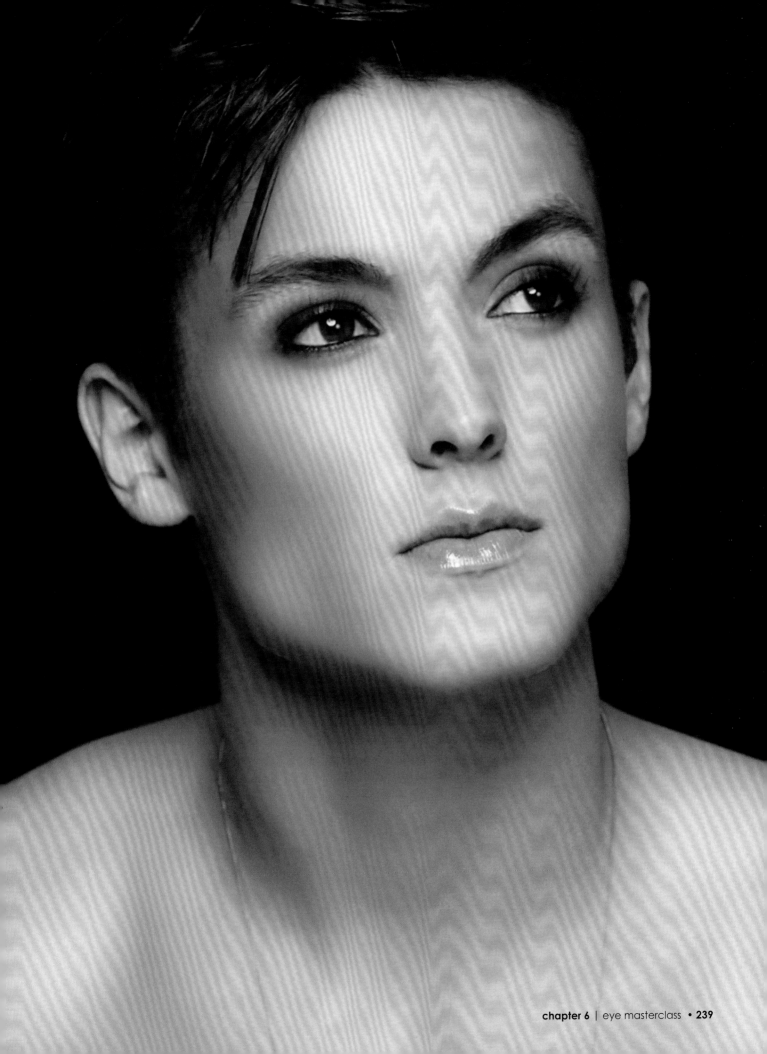

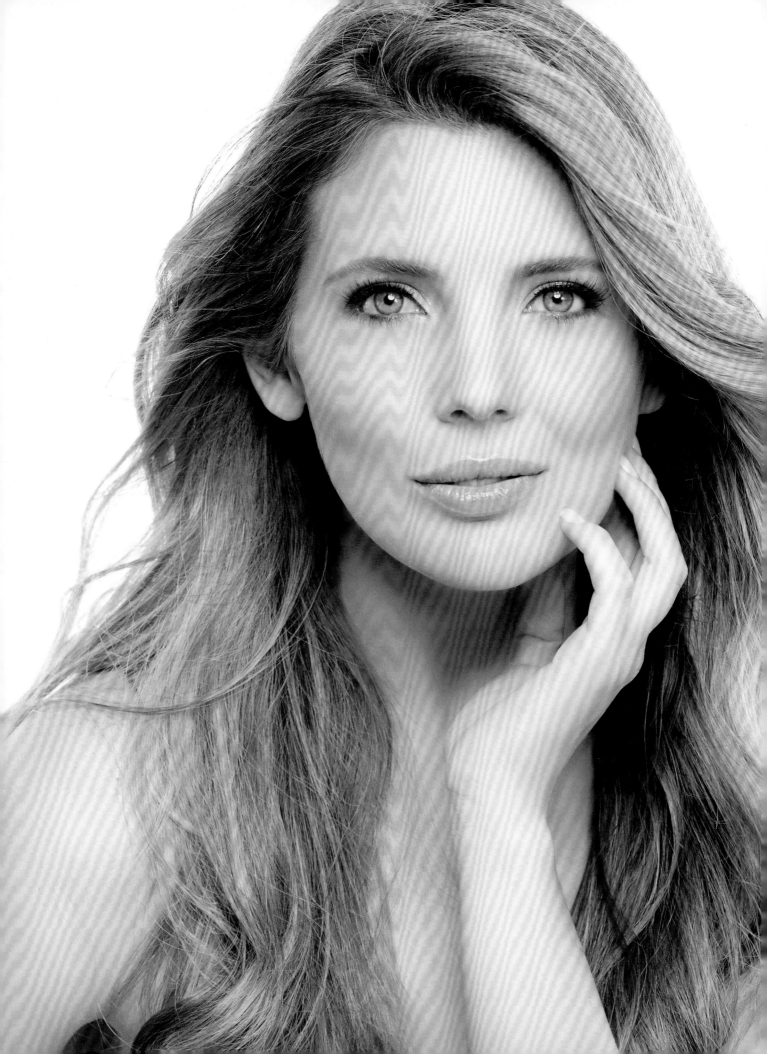

chapter 7

getting cheeky

A lot of people walk around with nothing on their cheeks. But for me, you're never finished without a little color. It goes such a long way toward bringing life to the face. I can't imagine finishing without some blush or bronzer. Everyone needs that last shot of color.

So why is it so often left out? Perhaps people don't understand why and how to use blush and bronzer. It's not about contouring with blush, and it's not about making you look tan with bronzer. Instead, it's about letting the products work together to create the perfect glow. Fortunately, you can get that glow simply and beautifully. Let's explore color and placement.

choose the right bronzer

Our goal with bronzer is not to make you look like you have a tan; it is just to give the skin a beautiful hint of color. Thus, you do not need one that is a great deal darker than your skin, just a shade or two darker. It should never be more than three shades darker than your skin's natural color.

For most people, the hardest part of picking out a bronzer is choosing the right shade. If you have ivory skin, choose one with a neutral tone; it should be more flesh toned, with a slight peach or pink undertone to it. If you have beige skin, you can use a little more of a golden tan undertone, which is perfect for your warm glow. And if you have ivory or beige skin, steer clear of orange. Too many of the products out there are far too orange, and there's nothing worse than a bright orange, overly bronzed face.

If you have olive (darker beige) skin, a bronzer with a saturated terra cotta or neutral brown undertone will give you the color you need. And if you have bronze or ebony skin, an intense copper or rich warm brown works best. Keep in mind that with dark ebony skin, your bronzer is not supposed to deepen your skin color. You already have beautiful rich depth to your skin, so just look for something with a slight shimmer to give you a glow.

Bronzers with a matte finish will always look the most natural on ivory or beige skin. I recommend a matte finish during the day. For a nighttime look with a little extra glow, you could add a layer with a little shimmer in it, but always start with a matte bronzer.

If you have light bronze skin, I would still, in most cases, recommend a bronzer with a matte finish because it gives the most natural effect. But if you have darker bronze to ebony skin, you need a little shimmer in your bronzer. If the finish is too matte, it can appear ashy on your skin. It doesn't have to be heavy on the shimmer—that could be too much even on dark skin—but a light shimmer will give you the glow you are looking for.

I have tried every shade of bronzer I can find, and they all look fake and too intense. You say I need one for a glow. What are my options?

If you feel that most bronzers are too heavily pigmented and give much more intense color than you want, try using a pressed powder instead. If you have ivory/beige skin, a bronze/ebony skin tone pressed powder will work wonderfully as a bronzer. It contains fewer pigments, helping it blend beautifully and look soft, subtle, and natural. You'll still get your glow—it will just be toned down a notch.

at first blush

One of the biggest makeup mistakes you can make is contouring with blush. You already know how to contour your face (see pages 92 and 101). Blush, meanwhile, is used to give the face color and life.

First, I want to dispel some of the old myths about placement:

Myth #1: Blush should never be worn closer to your nose than the width of two fingers. This rule might not work for everyone. Depending on the width of your fingers, your blush could end up on the side of your face instead of coming all the way to the apples of your cheeks!

Myth #2: Blush should never be applied to your cheek below the tip of your nose. If you follow this advice and you have a cute little turned-up nose, your blush could be applied above the apples of your cheeks (on top of your cheekbones). This certainly does not work for everyone.

Myth #3: As you age, you should apply cheek color higher. Although your skin may lose some of its elasticity as you age, I can assure you that your cheekbones remain in the same place!

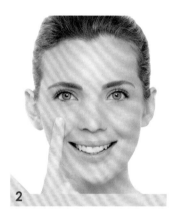

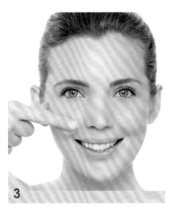

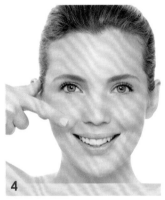

Forget the old myths. When applying bronzer and blush, you want to concentrate most of your color on the cheekbone. Where exactly is your cheekbone? No worries—it's easy to find. Just take this can't-miss application placement test:

1. Smile.

2. Locate the center of the "apple" of your cheek and place your index finger there.

3. Place your thumb at the top of your ear where it connects to your head.

4. Now, take your thumb and bring it toward your index finger. The bone you feel is your cheekbone.

5. Apply the color directly onto your cheekbone.

how to apply bronzer

Bronzer makes your skin look sun-kissed and alive. It gives it a healthy glow without subjecting it to damaging ultraviolet rays. To warm your face and accentuate your bone structure, simply dust bronzing powder or crème bronzer along your cheekbones, the outer edges of your face, and your temples. Bronzer is also useful for lightly sculpting the nose and defining your jawline and chin (see pages 97–98 and 103–104).

powder

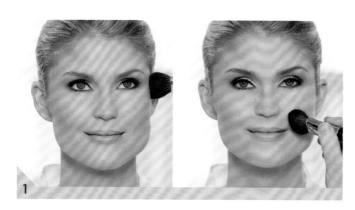

1. Make sure you have a nice, fluffy, full bronzer brush; this will help with your blending and give you the most natural application. Begin at the back of your cheekbone and sweep the bronzer forward toward the apple of your cheek. Then take the brush back toward your ear. This lays your color in place.

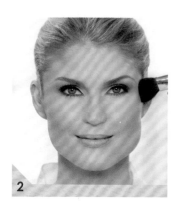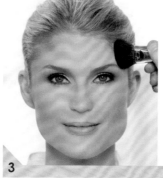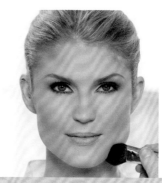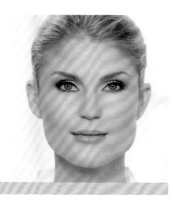

2. Use the brush in the opposite direction (up and down) to blend. Blend well.

3. Add a little bronzer at your temples to help shape your face. Sweeping the bronzing powder up around the temples and eye sockets can also help your eye color pop, especially if your eyes are green or blue. Finish by sweeping your bronzer along your jawline to add definition.

crème and gel

1. With your finger or a sponge, dot the color all along your cheekbone. Start at the apple of your cheek and work toward your ear.

3. Blend a little up onto your temples for the ultimate glow.

2. With a clean finger or sponge, blend the color out (up and down) and back toward your ear.

how to apply blush

Using blush is about adding a beautiful shot of color to your face, giving it life. It's the perfect way to add color back to your face as you age, but also just a great way to add a great glow at any age. You have multiple options when come to how to get it.

powder

A powder blush is the easiest to use. Just as with bronzer, make sure to use a soft, full brush for your best application; it will help you achieve the most natural and blended look. There are two ways to apply your powder blush: a basic method that gives you more intense color and a technique called "popping your apples" that will give you a very soft, natural flush.

basic method

1. For the most color, apply blush to your cheekbone area, starting at the back (closest to your ear). Sweep your cheek color toward the apple of your cheek and then back toward the ear again. This lays your color in place.

2. Use the brush in the opposite direction (up and down) to blend. The most intense color will lie at the back of your cheeks, giving your face more dimension.

apple popping method

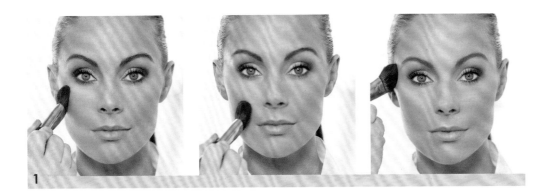

1. Apply bronzer to your cheekbones, starting at the back (closest to your ear). Sweep your cheek color toward the apple of your cheek and then back toward the ear again. This lays your color in place.

2. Use the brush in the opposite direction (up and down) to blend.

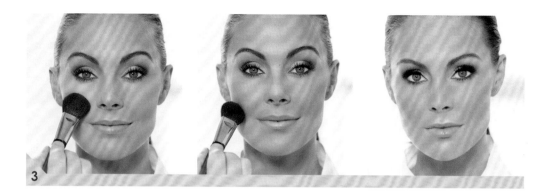

3. Now grab a light, sheer, colorful blush. Smile and apply your blush color to the apples of your cheeks, blending back toward the area that you bronzed. This gives the apples of your cheeks, where the color is concentrated, a beautiful glow. The secret is color selection; you'll want to use a sheer shade of blush because a dark or intense cheek color can be too harsh and unnatural-looking when applied this way. Your goal is to glow, not to paint Raggedy Ann–style circles on your cheeks.

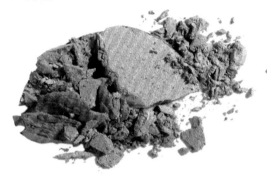

Q & A

I have tried everything—crème, powder, and liquid blush. Nothing stays on! My skin seems to absorb it all. What can I do to keep color on my face?

Increase wear-ability and the intensity of the color by layering your blush. It should last all day.

1. After applying your foundation, apply a crème blush to the apples of your cheeks and cheekbones.

2. Dust your face with loose or pressed powder.

3. Apply a powder blush (similar in color to the crème blush) to the apples of your cheeks and cheekbones.

crème or liquid blush

If you use crème or liquid blush, apply it with a sponge, your fingers, or a crème blush brush after your foundation and before your powder for easier blending. If you wear your blush without foundation, crème and liquid work better than powder blush because they contain moisture that blends better with the natural moisture of your skin.

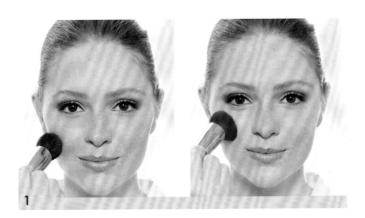

1. To apply crème or liquid blush, first dot a little onto the apples of your cheeks.

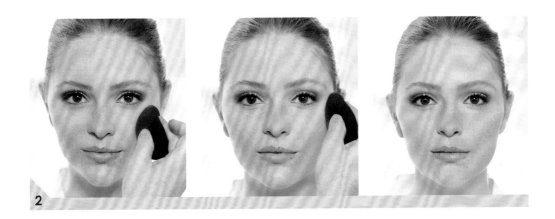

2. Then blend back toward your ears with a clean sponge.

With any blush, you should remember this rule: Always match textures—crème on crème and powder on powder. Apply crème or liquid blush after your foundation and before your powder. If you wait until after you powder, it will not go on smoothly or evenly. Apply powder blush after your foundation and powder; if you apply it before you powder, it will go on splotchy and uneven.

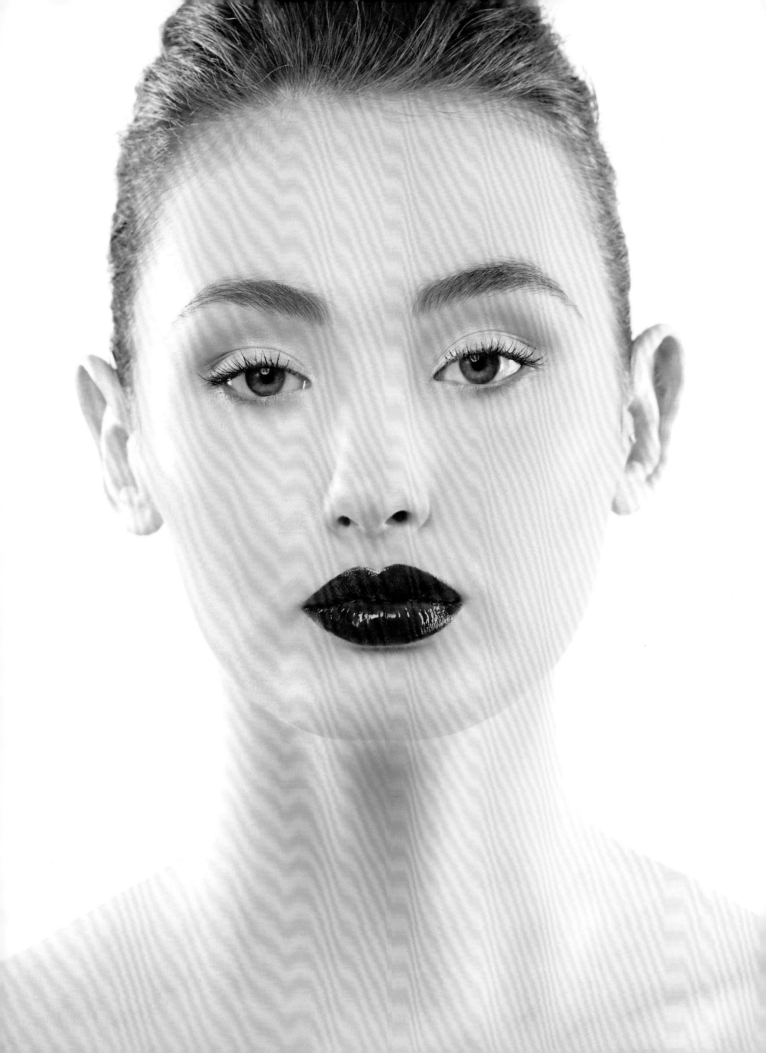

chapter 8

pout perfect

Who wouldn't love to walk around with stunningly beautiful, full lips? It's entirely possible, but a lot goes into getting the perfect pout. First, we've already talked about the importance of picking the right color. Color can make a big impact, so choose carefully. Then we can start to talk about application and technique.

Lip liner and lipstick are great tools for creating effects. You can create shading on red or nude lips that take them to a whole new level. The right shade of liner can ground a shade that feels a bit too bright. With the right lip liner and lipstick, you can create a gradation of color that will give the illusion of fullness or even add depth. The right combination of colors and techniques can be life changing.

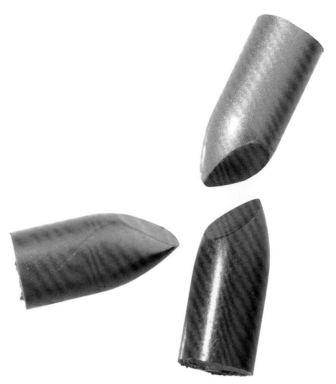

lip service

To keep your lips looking luscious and because color adheres better to a smooth surface, exfoliate your lips at least once a week. To exfoliate, simply apply a generous layer of lip balm to your lips, let it soak in for a few minutes, and then brush your lips with a soft baby's toothbrush. (You could even brush them while you are brushing your teeth.) Rub them with a nubby-textured washcloth if you don't have a toothbrush handy. The balm will soften the dry skin so that brushing or rubbing them will remove the dry layer of skin, leaving the lips soft and smooth.

I always like to use a little lip balm or moisturizer on the lips before I apply lip color, because it helps the lip liner and lipstick go on smoothly and more evenly. Just apply the lip balm when you first start doing your make-up, at the same time you apply your moisturizer. This will give the balm time to soak in. Then, right before you apply your lip color, blot off the excess so the balm won't shorten your lip color's wearing time.

apply lip liner

Lining your lips with lip pencil will help prevent lipstick from feathering and bleeding, but don't stop there. Be sure to blend inward so that when your lipstick wears off, you aren't left with just an outline. Your lip liner should never be visible after you have applied your lipstick and/or gloss. You'll find that a lip brush will help give you a more precise application and help everything blend better.

Make sure to optimize your entire mouth. Most people don't; they tend to draw inside their natural lip line. Most of the time, your lip line extends farther than the colored portion of the lip. Use your entire lip!

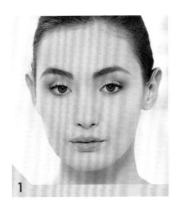

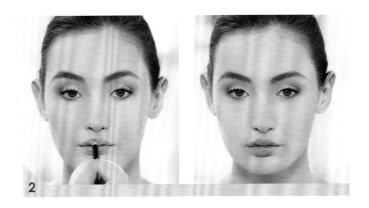

1. Optional: Use concealer or foundation to conceal your natural lip line, which creates a perfect canvas to draw back on your lip line.

2. Begin with a letter v in your "cupid's bow," or the center curve of your lips. Bring the liner up and around the curves of your bow.

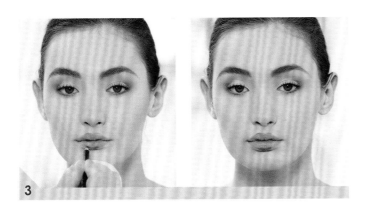

3. Accentuate the lower curve of your lower lip.

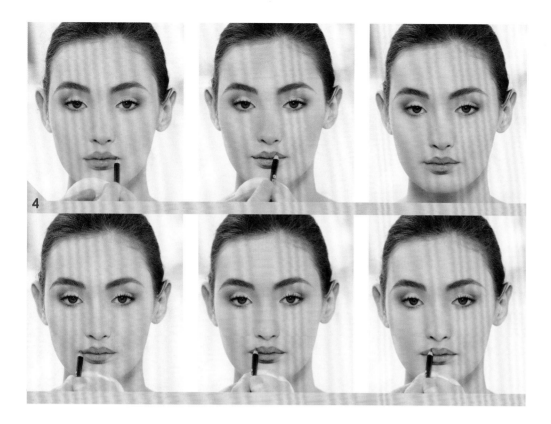

4. Starting at the outer corners, bring your pencil toward the center bow, connecting the lines. Repeat with the other side.

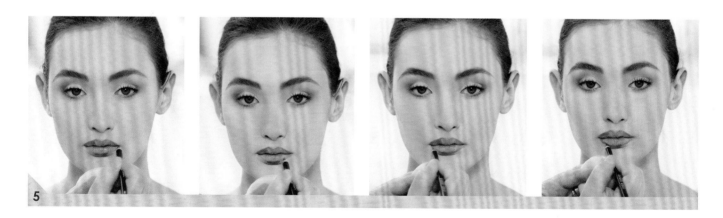

5. Starting in the outside corner of your lower lip, bring your pencil toward the center, connecting your lines. Repeat on the other side.

tip: *To keep your lipstick from traveling, choose an intense shade and dab it on with your finger, using very little product.*

6. Remember to use your entire lip: Take the color to the nearly invisible line at the edge of the colored part of your lips. Blend with a lip brush to make it look its most natural.

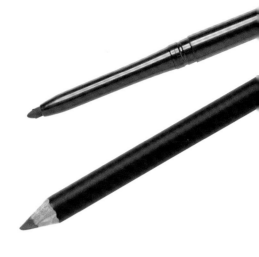

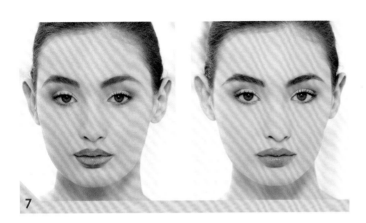

7

7. Your lips are now ready for lipstick and gloss.

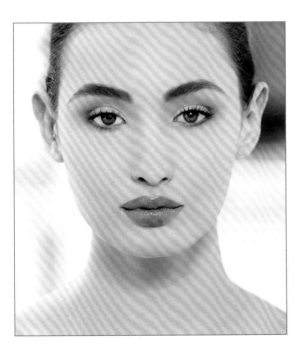

You can use a brush, your fingers, or a tube to apply your lipstick, but if it's applied with a brush, it will usually look much more precise and last longer. For more intense color, you can apply it straight from the tube, but it will be harder to cover the smaller, detailed areas of your lips. Even if you do apply it straight from the tube, you could go back over it with a brush for a better blend. Similarly, if you apply your lip gloss with a brush, it will appear shinier than if you apply it with a sponge tip.

tip: *Putting on lipstick straight from the tube will not blend your lip liner. You should always blend your lip liner with a brush toward the center of the lips.*

tip: *To keep lipstick from smearing onto your teeth, after application, stick your finger in your mouth and pull it out. This will remove any color on the inside of your lips, so it won't smear onto your teeth.*

Do I have to wear lip liner?

No, but it does three things for you:

1. It helps define your mouth and reshape your lips if they are uneven, giving them a nice edge.

2. It helps prevent your lip color from bleeding.

3. It helps your lipstick last longer, especially if you fill in your lips. I always fill in at least halfway toward the center of the mouth with lip liner before I apply lipstick.

I never know which lip liner I should choose. Should my lip liner be darker than my lipstick, the same color, or what?

You never want your lip liner to be darker than your lipstick. (If it is, make sure to fill in your entire lip before applying your lip color so it doesn't look like you just ate an Oreo cookie.) A shade the same as your natural lips will always work, no matter what shade you apply on top, because it will match your natural coloring. Keep in mind, though, your liner color can change your lipstick or gloss shade. For example, if you are using a bright shade, it could mute the color, and if you are using a deep shade, it could lighten it. If you choose a bright lip color you don't want muted or softened, choose a lip liner that matches your lipstick or gloss. If you choose a deep lip color you don't want lightened, choose a shade that matches your lipstick or lip gloss in depth.

It seems that no matter what shade I choose, it shifts color on me and turns pink. What is happening and can I prevent it?

If your skin's pH is highly alkaline, the alkalinity in your skin can react with the lipstick pigment and cause it to shift to a pink or orange color. You can't stop it from happening, but you can prevent a strong color shift by using the opposite color. For instance, if your skin shifts everything pink, a shade that has a lot of warmth (orange) in it will shift more neutral. And if you shift everything orange, a shade with a lot of pink in it will shift more neutral and less orange. Where a neutral shade can shift one way or the other, if you start out with the complete opposite, it will not be able to shift all the way to the shade you are trying to prevent. You can use either lip liner or lipstick to prevent the color shift or layer the two.

My lip color never lasts. How can I get longer wear out of it?

This method works best and keeps your lips feeling their most supple.

1. Conceal the entire lip area, everything from your natural lip line to your actual lips.

2. Line the outer edges of your lips with lip liner and then fill in the entire lip area with liner (use the side of the pencil rather than the point for a more even application of color). This is the first line of defense in getting your lip color to last. Lip liner has a drier texture than lipstick, so it lasts longer.

3. Apply your lipstick and then take a tissue and gently blot your lips. This will remove the moisture from this layer, yet leave you with a deposit of lipstick pigment.

4. Reapply your lipstick; this time, do not blot. The double pigment deposit increases how long the color will wear.

5. Finish with a dot of lip gloss in the center of your lips.

It seems that no matter what I wear, lipstick or lip gloss, it bleeds. Is there any way to prevent my lip color from bleeding?

You want to create a dam (or ledge) so nothing can bleed outward. You will also need to fill in any fine lines around your mouth. Here are some of the products and techniques to consider:

1. Use lip liner; it is your first line of defense to prevent bleeding.

2. Dip a Q-tip into loose powder and run it all along the outer edge of your lip.

3. With your concealer brush, apply a dab of concealer all around your mouth just at the edge of the lip line. This will create a great dam while filling in any fine lines you might have. This is one of the most effective ways to prevent bleeding without buying any additional products.

4. You can purchase products designed to create a dam (or ledge) for you. They have a waxy, velvety texture. They're clear, so they never show. Apply one all around the outer edge of your lip.

5. If you do not want to take any extra steps, apply less lipstick so it won't slide and bleed. Instead of applying your lipstick with a brush or the tube, simply dab it on with your fingers. This will apply the lightest possible layer, just a stain on your lips rather than a full layer of lipstick.

fuller lips

One of the makeup effects with the biggest bang is making your lips look fuller. Not only do most people with thinner lips want their lips to look fuller, but fuller lips make you look younger, softer, and even friendlier. As we age, our lips lose some of their fullness, so this technique can come in handy. You need three tools to make this happen: a natural tone lip liner, a natural tone lipstick (if it is too dark it will only make your lips look smaller), and a shimmering lip gloss. It's easy and effective, so let's give it a try:

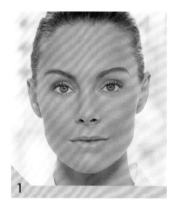

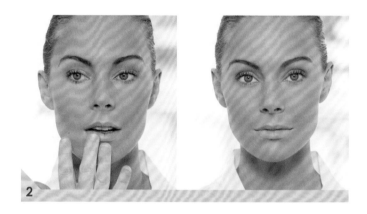

1. Exfoliate and moisturize your lips with lip balm to make sure they are smooth and ready for color.

2. Erase your existing lip line with concealer or foundation, creating a fresh canvas on which you can create your new improved lip.

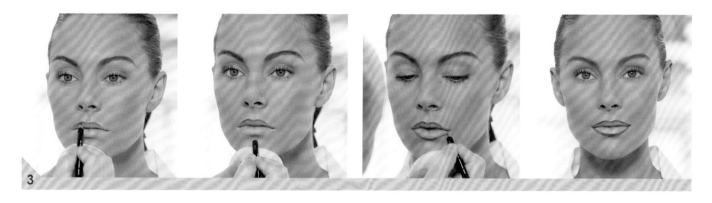

3. Using a natural-toned lip pencil (not dark, but neutral and natural), draw a line just slightly above your natural lip across the top and slightly below your lip along your lower lip line. Don't exaggerate the line.

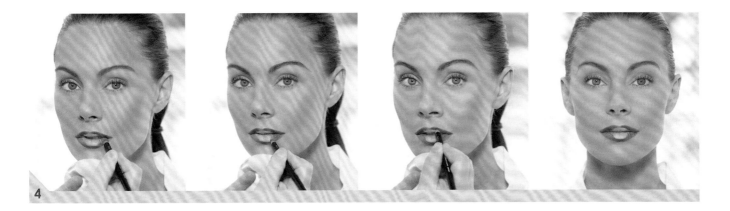

4. Fill in your lips with lip liner, except for the very centers of your top and bottom lips.

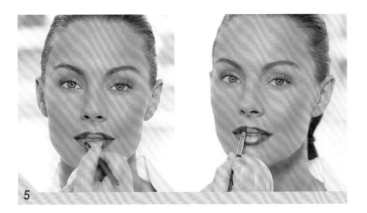

5. Using a lip brush, blend in your lip liner.

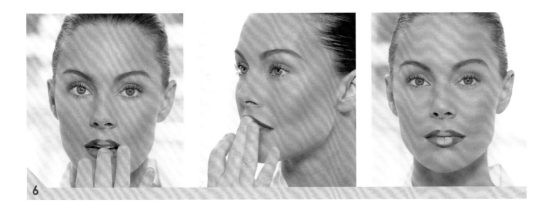

6. Place a dab of concealer in the centers of your top and bottom lips.

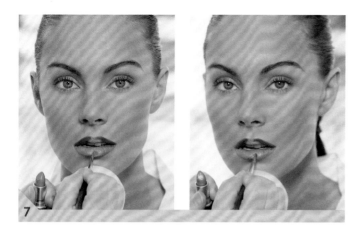

7. Apply your lipstick. It will mix with the concealer, keeping the center of your lips lighter and making them appear fuller.

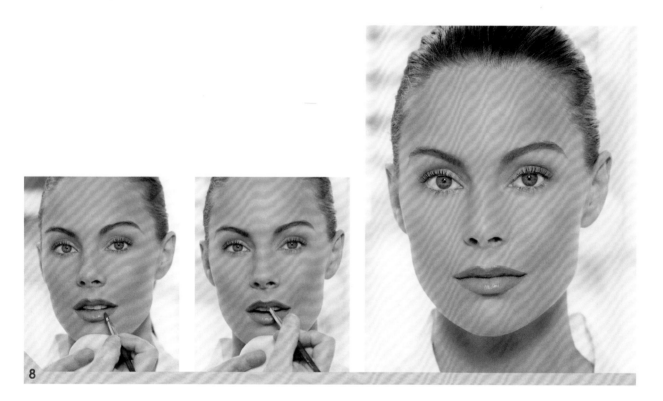

8. To finish, apply a light, shimmery lip gloss to the center of your lips over your lipstick (blending it outward). This will reflect light, helping your lips appear even fuller.

tip: *For the most natural-looking lipstick, choose a shade close to your own lip color, just glossier and slightly deeper.*

the perfect red lip

Creating the perfect red lip is all about grounding it because most red lipsticks tend to glow on the face without the grounding. You need a gradation of darkness on the outer edges slowly moving to a lighter red on the interiors. This not only makes the lip look fuller, but it gives the red lip a nice edge.

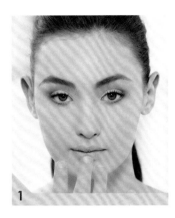

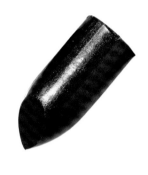

1. Exfoliate and moisturize your lips with lip balm to make sure they are smooth and ready for color.

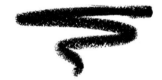

2. Erase your existing lip line with concealer or foundation.

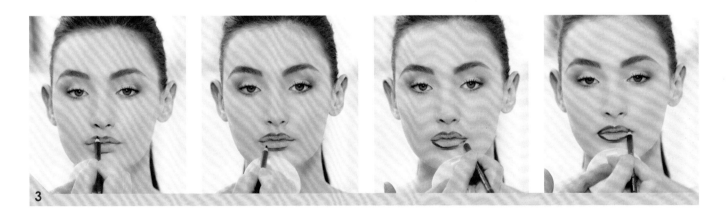

3. Using a burgundy (or if you prefer, chocolate) lip liner, line your lips.

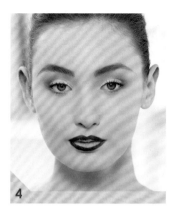

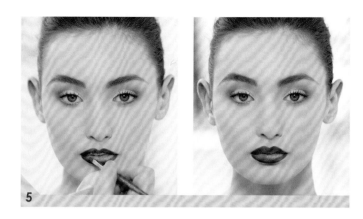

4. Now fill in your lips with that same lip liner, except for the center. This will create more depth in the outer edge of your lip while keeping the center slightly lighter.

5. Using a lip brush, blend in your lip liner.

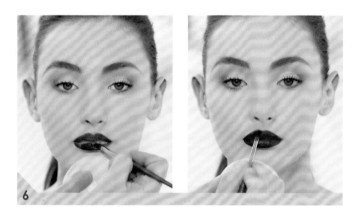

6. With a lip brush for an exact application, apply your favorite red lipstick. Start in the center and work toward the edges so you can get an exact edge. You can always go back with a concealer brush and some concealer and fix the edge if you make a mistake.

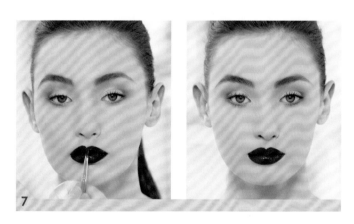

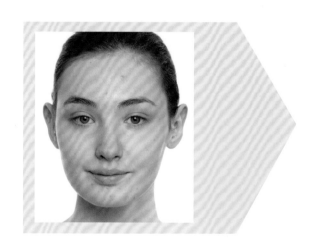

7. Finish with red or burgundy gloss, depending on the effect you want. Start your application in the center of the lip and keep the majority of the product there to help prevent bleeding.

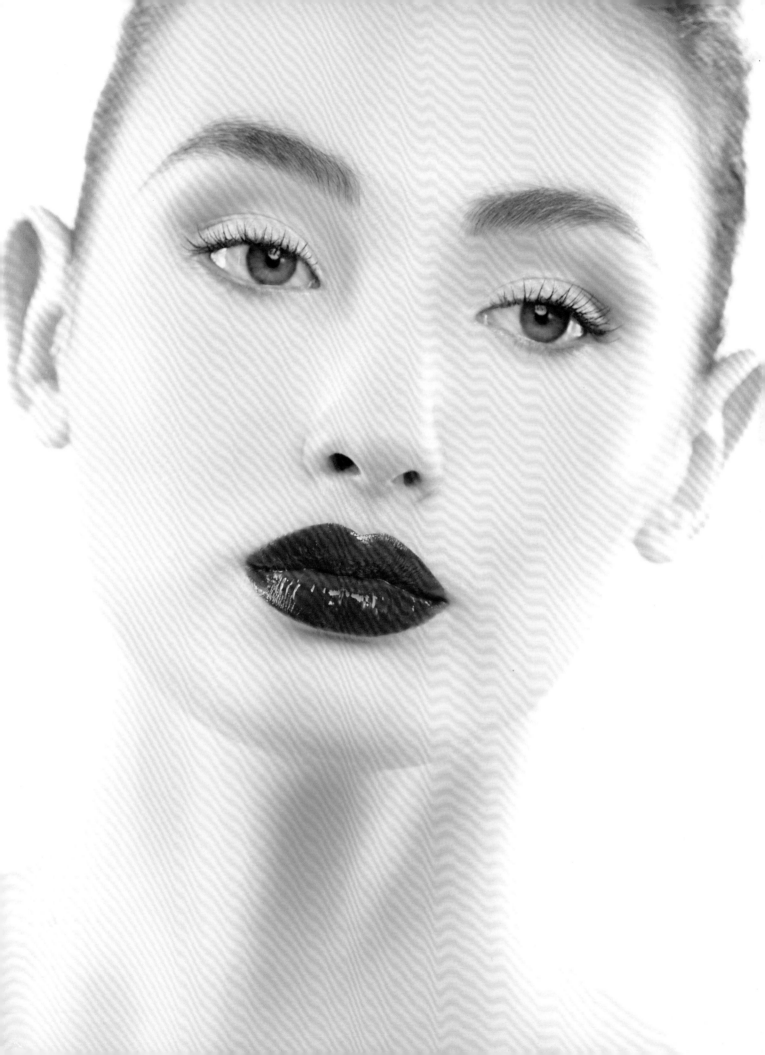

the perfect nude lip

Most people think the perfect nude lip is just about choosing the right shade, but it also requires the right application. Because it is such a pale color, it is about creating a gradation of color. It's about creating a little bit more depth in the outer edge of the lip for definition.

Picking the exact shade you need may seem daunting, but with the right one, everyone looks great in a nude lip. If you have ivory skin, pick a shade with some pink or peach in it; anything too beige could make you look too washed out. If you have beige to dark beige skin, look for a nude with a peach, beige, or caramel tone. And if you have bronze or ebony skin, look for a nude with deep caramel and mocha tones for the perfect pucker.

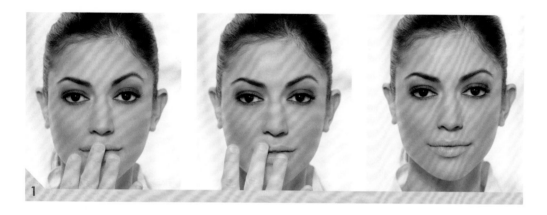

1. Exfoliate and moisturize your lips with lip balm to make sure they are smooth and ready for all color.

2. Erase your existing lip line with concealer or foundation.

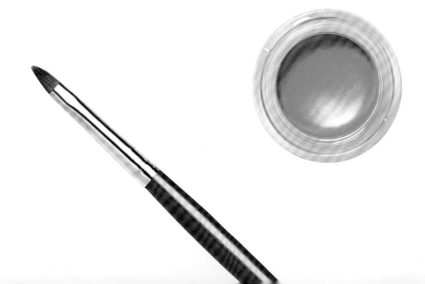

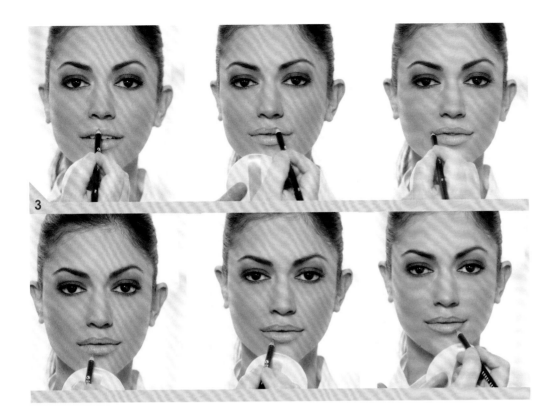

3. Using a nude lip liner that is one level deeper than your lipstick, line your lips.

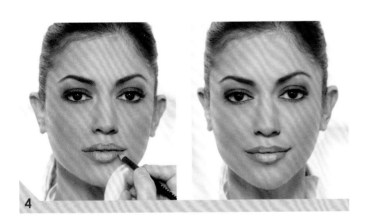
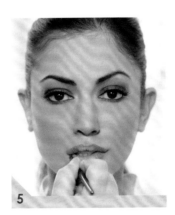

4. Using the same lip liner, fill in all but the centers of your upper and lower lips.

5. Using a lip brush, blend in your lip liner.

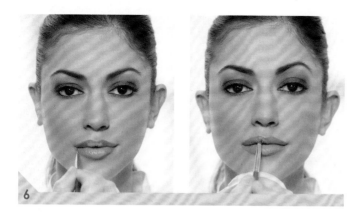

6. With your lip brush for exact application, apply your favorite nude lipstick.

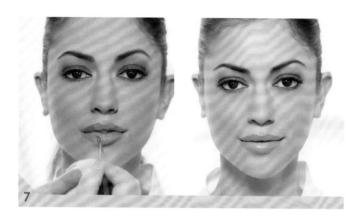

7. Finish with nude lip gloss for extra shine and shape.

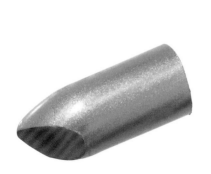

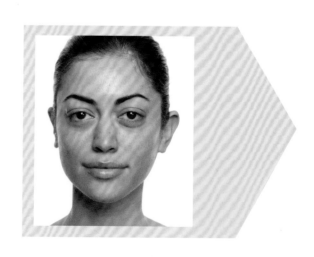

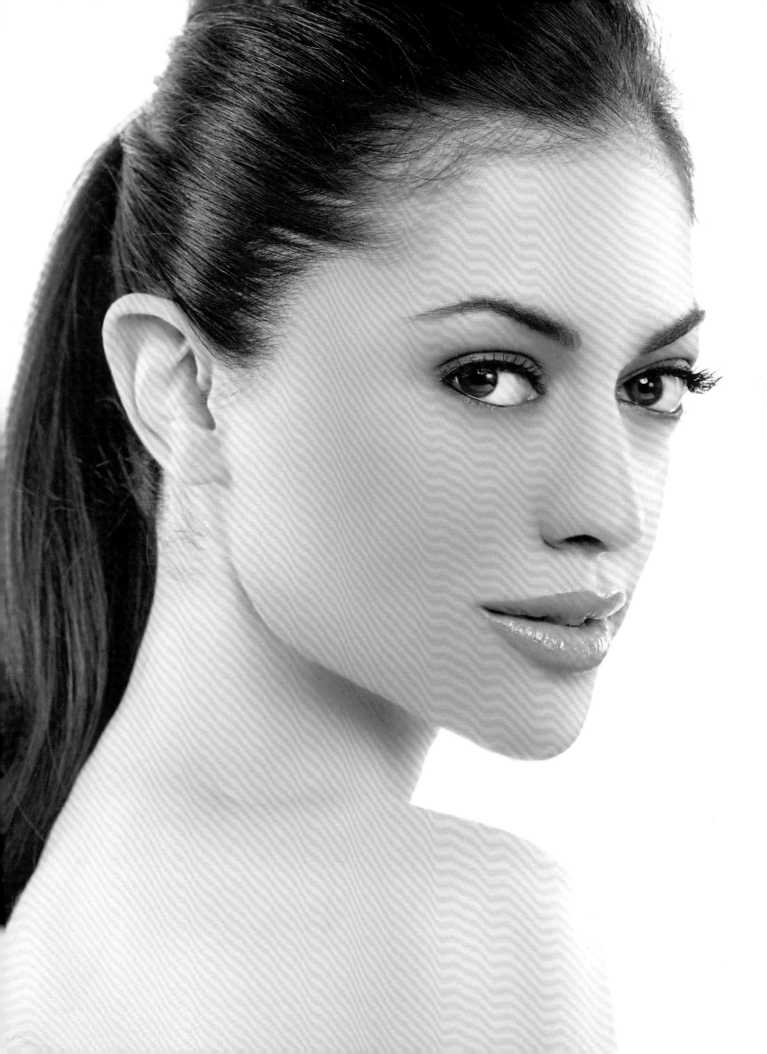

chapter 9

beauty at any age

For many, the quests for beauty and youth go hand in hand. Many of the techniques we have already learned will go a long way toward making you look younger. Maybe that means pushing back a hooded lid or shaping your lid to look its absolute best. Maybe it's making great color choices to bring life and color to your face. Maybe it's mastering highlighting and contouring, which are especially good at giving you an impressively youthful glow.

There are a few other considerations that will also help us in our quest for youth. Let's talk about some of the other things we need to think about to look younger, specifically skin, lips, and eyes.

your skin as you age

As we age, our skin constantly changes. Most people's skin gets drier, so you will need to moisturize more than you ever have. Even if you have oily skin, it won't be as oily as it once was. An even, flawless complexion always makes you look younger, and moisture is a big part of that. You may also want to move to a foundation with added hydration. It's not a must for everyone, but it can be helpful.

You may also find that you need less powder. I'm not saying you will stop using it completely, but because your skin is drier and you might have more fine lines, you may discover you need less. You will still need to use it to set your foundation and concealer so they will last all day, but you might find you need less to do the job.

your eyes as you age

You don't have to change a lot to stay looking youthful when it comes to eye makeup. Update your look regularly, but you don't have to stop wearing eye makeup. In fact, that could age you.

As you get older, your lids may become dry or crepey. But don't apply moisturizer or eye crème to your eyelids before you put on eye shadow because it will cause it to crease and not last as long. If you want to moisturize your lids, do it before bed, not in the morning.

If you have always worn eyeliner, you should continue to line your eyes; maybe just make a softer shade choice. Actually, eyeliner can go a long way toward helping to define your eyes (opening them up and drawing attention to them). Some women think they should stop wearing eyeliner as they age, but that's just not true. All you have to do is make better color choices. For example, if you wore black eyeliner in your twenties, switch to brown to create a softer, more youthful definition in your fifties. If you think your brown is now too intense, switch to a soft bronze or taupe. Don't stop defining your eyes as you age; just soften the definition.

With eye shadows, you might want to move away from frosts and toward shimmers as you age and your eyelids get crepey. When they get more crepey, move to strictly matte eye shadows so they won't draw any attention to the texture. It's all about choices, this time involving color *and texture*.

When we age, our eyelashes tend to thin out, and that can show age. Anything you can do to make your eyelashes to look fuller will make your eyes look more youthful. That could mean a couple more layers of mascara or added eyelashes.

tip: *You might want to use more waterproof or water-resistant products, including eyeliner and mascara, because as we age we tend to have more issues with eyes watering.*

I need concealer under my eyes to cover up some darkness, but it draws attention to my fine lines. What can I do?

Moisturize with an eye crème, which will help keep the skin supple. Also, make your concealer more moisturizing by mixing it with your eye crème before you apply it.

I conceal under my eyes, and when I'm finished it looks great, but when I powder to set it, which I know I need to do, it accentuates lines and texture. What can I do?

Use the finger powder method: Dip your clean finger in some loose powder, rub the excess off in your palm, and trace it over the area you need to powder. That should set it without drawing attention to fine lines. If you have just finished powdering under your eyes and it looks a little dry and caked, lightly pat on a tiny bit of eye crème. Don't rub or work it in. Leave it alone after you pat it on; just let it melt in.

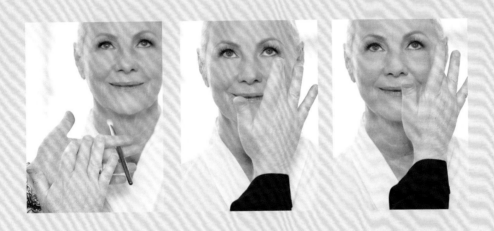

As I go through my day, the skin under my eyes starts to appear dry and crepey. What can I do?

Moisturize as frequently as you like! Lightly pat a tiny bit of eye crème over the area. Don't rub it in, just let it melt in. This will rehydrate the area.

I have very dry skin. Do I still need to powder my face?

Absolutely! You may not need to powder your whole face, but even people with dry skin need to powder their T-zone area (the center of the face, forehead, nose, front of the cheeks, and tip of the chin) to cut the shine.

My brows have thinned out over the years. Is it true that fuller brows make you look younger? How can I make them look fuller, but still natural?

Yes, fuller brows do make you look younger, and brows do thin naturally as you age. Part of that is that they don't remain as high as they used to, and as they drop, they thin out (just my own personal theory). You can add a bit of fullness back by layering pencil and powder. This will give you more coverage, look more natural, and help the color last longer (see page 118).

I am not letting my hair go gray, but I am starting to get flecks of gray in my eyebrows. I try to cover them with pencil and powder, and nothing really covers the gray. If I tweeze them, my brows are too sparse. Do I have any other option for covering gray hairs in my brows?

Yes—you can have them professionally tinted. There are special and specific tints that are just for the eye area, and tinting the brows will completely cover the gray hairs. But, please, have this done by a professional who knows what they are doing. Do not do it yourself at home!

your lips as you age

As we age, our lips lose volume. Keep that in mind especially if you have ivory or beige skin. Dark shades will age you and make your lips look even smaller, so keep that in mind when choosing your shade.

Adding back a little color can go a long way toward adding a little life back to your face. It doesn't have to be super bright, just a nice shot of a little warm color. Revisit your color theory (see page 45) for your best color choices.

Last, because your lips, just like the rest of your skin, tend to be drier as you age, think about choosing formulas that add a lot of moisture. This will make your lips look much more supple and full. Don't be afraid to wear lip gloss; that always adds the look of fullness. You might also want to try the fuller lip technique (see page 256). You may also find more fine lines around your lips, which could cause your lipstick and gloss to be more likely to bleed (to stop this from happening, see the Q & A on page 255).

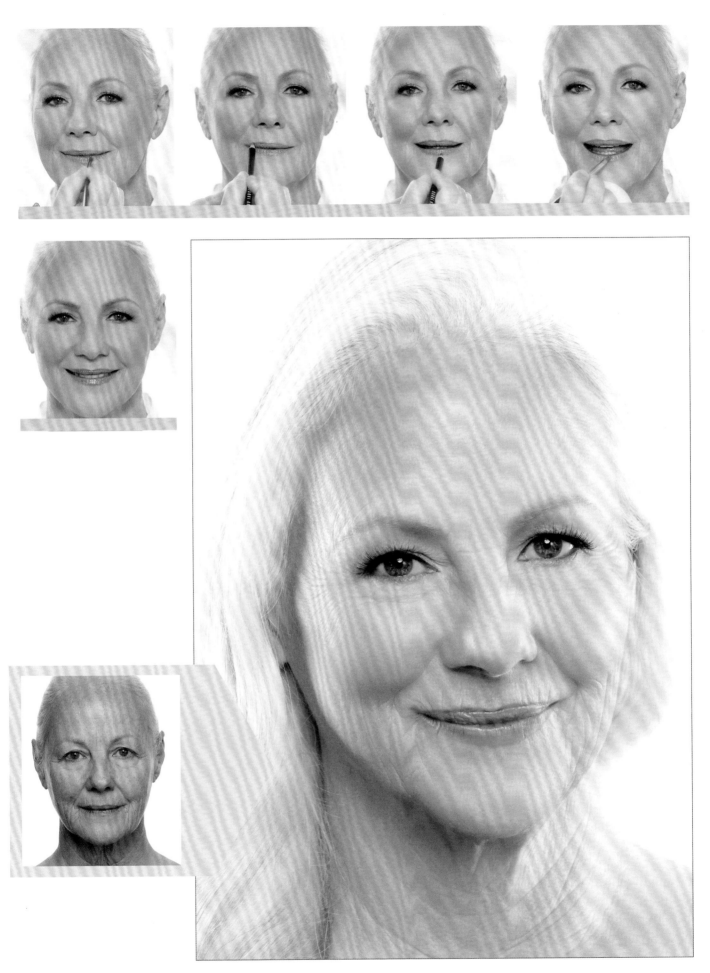

blush/bronzer as you age

Blush and bronzer are probably your best friends when it comes to looking younger. Adding color back to you skin will always make you look younger. As we age, the first thing that happens is that we lose pigment and tone in our skin, making us look washed out. Adding back that color adds life and a glow back to your face. It can easily take ten years off.

Just make sure, as always, that you make the correct shade choices. Remember that warm blush shades will always make you look younger than cool blush shades will. Review your color theory (see page 45) to help you pick your perfect youthful glow-enhancing color. You can see here what a difference the right bronzer and blush can make.

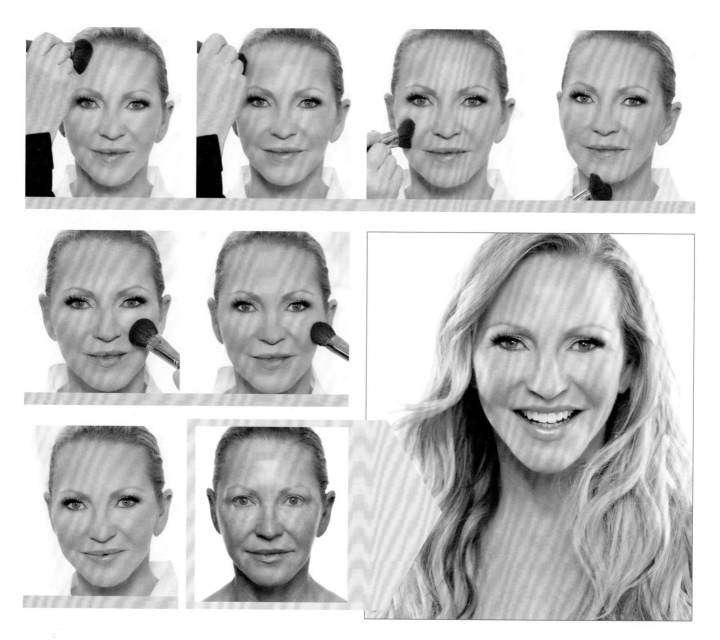

I have very dry skin, and when I wear powder blush it seems to just sit on top of my skin and doesn't look natural. What can I do?

For very dry skin, a crème or a gel blush is a much better choice. It is more moisturizing and will last longer and look much more natural. It blends into dry skin, while powder will just sit on top. Just remember that when using a crème or gel, apply it after foundation and before you powder (which, if you have dry skin, you will be doing very little of), or it will not go on evenly.

The definition along my jawline has softened and is less taut than it used to be, making me look older. What can I do to re-create that youthful definition?

One of the signs of aging that people object to most is the softening (a slight drooping of the skin) of their jawline. There is a quick, easy fix using make-up to re-create the definition of youth and make the droopy skin much less visible: After you have finished applying your makeup, use a narrow, slightly flat, dense brush and a matte bronzer (no shimmer; it will not look natural) to apply a light layer all along your jawline. This will create a little more definition (giving you back your youthful jawline) and make the droopy skin much less visible. Also, anytime there is an area of you face you do not like, it also helps to draw attention away from it to minimize it. For example, wearing a softer lip color and slightly more intense eye makeup will draw everyone's eyes up and away from the lower area of your face—whereas if you wore a dark or intense lip color, it would draw everyone's eyes to the area you don't want them to see. Many times, looking younger is all about concentrating on the features you love about your face.

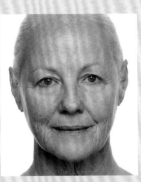
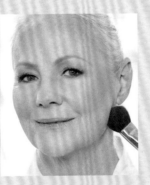

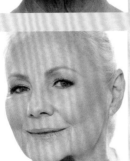
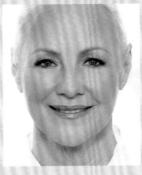

Q & A

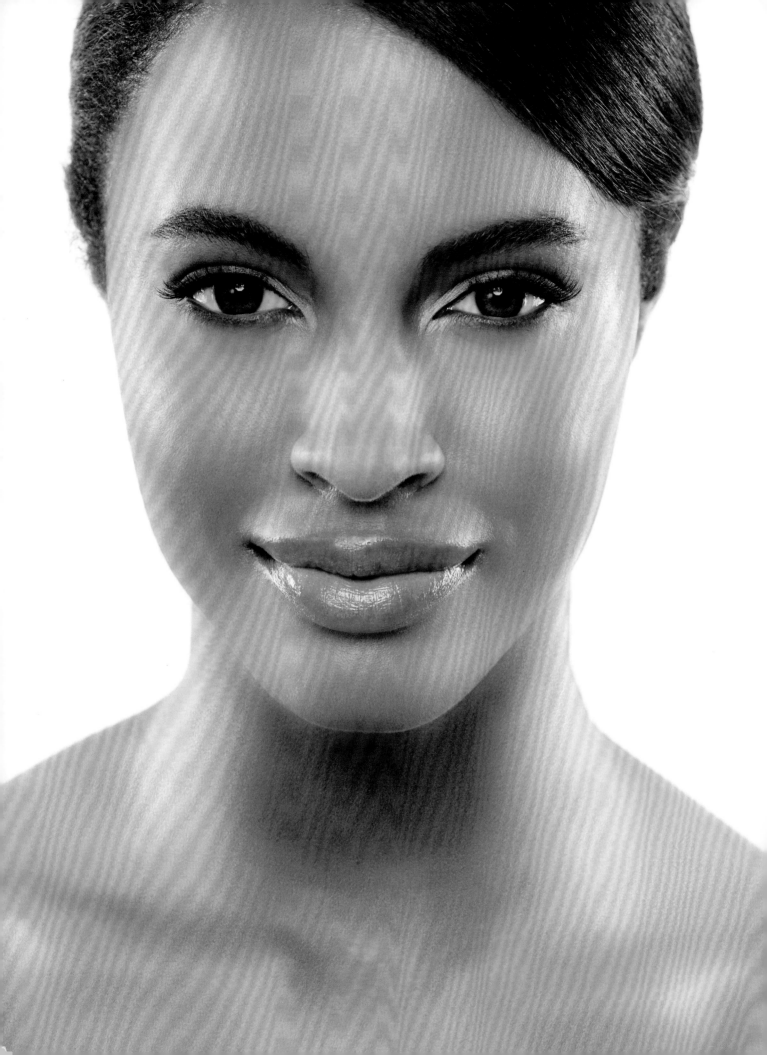

chapter 10

that
special day

In the end, the most important mementos of your wedding are the photographs, because fifteen years from now, when what you wore no longer fits, the one thing you are going to look back on are the photos. The time of day you get married, as well as the way you photograph at that time of day, will affect your makeup choices. For example, the natural look of a morning wedding varies greatly from the more dramatic look of an evening ceremony. The way the sunlight changes throughout the day can affect the way your makeup appears in photos. It can also affect the type of lighting your photographer will choose.

I divide brides into four categories, based on the time of day they're getting married: morning, midday, late afternoon, and evening. With each time choice, there are certain details you'll want to consider. Paying attention to them can help you get the best wedding photos possible.

morning bride

For a morning wedding, your makeup look should appear soft and pretty to match the cool, soft morning light. Morning light has a blue tint. Mornings are perfect for the natural girl; it's the time of day when a bride should wear the least amount of makeup. Most brides who get married in the morning have the event outside, or at least take their photos and portraits outside. Even if they are getting married inside, the photographer might be taking advantage of the light coming through windows rather than using a lot of artificial light for the photographs.

- Though a matte foundation is always perfect for photographs, a morning bride can choose to wear a foundation with a slight sheen or dewiness to it, because the light will be so soft. Make sure that your skin is a nice, even tone (see page 66).

- Make sure to prep you skin well so your foundation lasts throughout the ceremony and reception without needing a ton of touchups.

- If your skin tends to break out, I would not choose this time of day for your wedding, because you are going to want to wear as little foundation and concealer as possible, due to the softer natural light.

- Go light on the powder so your face retains its natural appearance. You want your skin to appear matte, but it does not take a lot of powder to achieve this. Heavy powder can appear artificial in the morning light.

- If you want, your blush can have a touch of shimmer to it at this time of day, because the photographer isn't likely to use a flash and the light is so soft. Just make sure you don't choose anything too bold.

- Don't make bold eyeshadow color choices for your eyes. Choose warmer, soft shades that complement your eye color. This is the one time you will want to wear less eyeshadow, because the lighting will accentuate any harsh colors or lack of blending.

- Define your eyes well at the lash line to help them stand out (see page 130). Another option would be false eyelashes (see page 188).

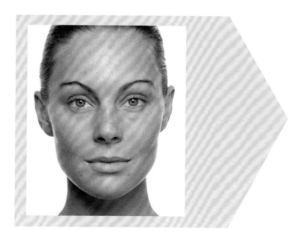

- If you choose to wear eyeliner (you don't have to), keep it subtle and soft. You don't want anything too dark (no black) or too harsh or thick—keep it really close to the lash line—at this time of day.

- Lip color should always be soft and natural—nothing too bold. If it is too bold, it will be all that you see in the photos.

- Everything will photograph darker than it appears to the eye, because the light is so soft, so go with softer shade choices.

- Make sure everything is well blended; any harsh lines or hard edges will just be magnified in the photos.

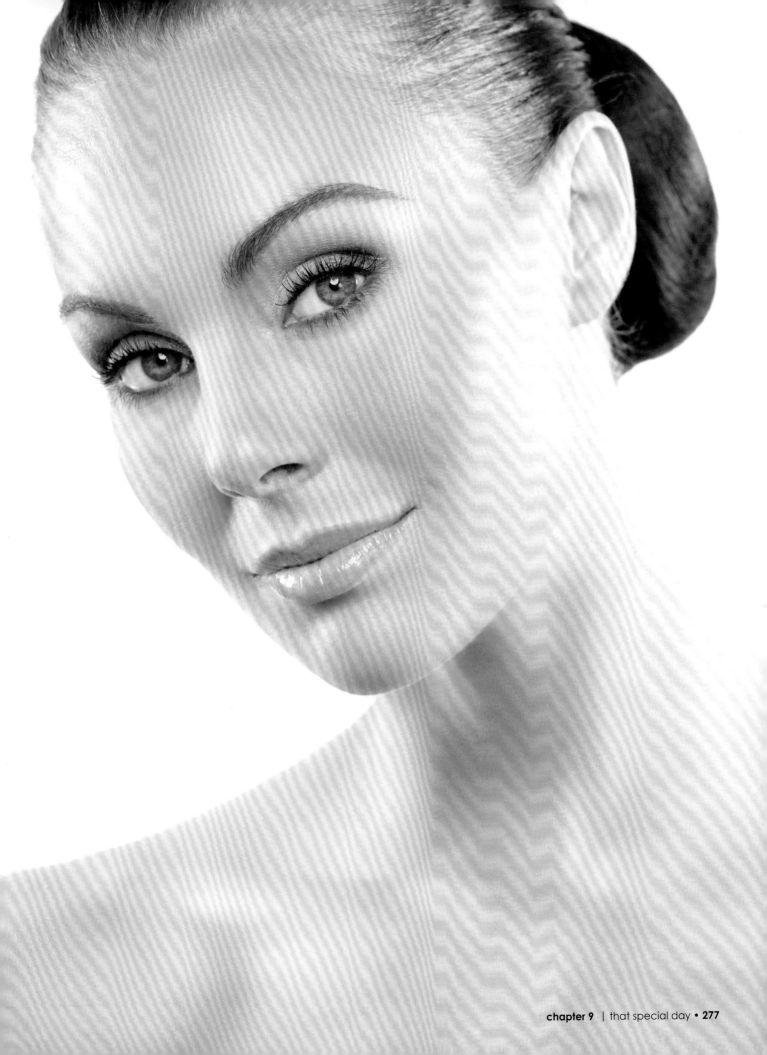

midday bride

If you're planning a wedding in the middle of the day, be aware that the midday sun can cast shadows on your face, which can make a difference if you're taking outdoor photos. This is the harshest light to be photographed in. Because the natural light will be coming from directly above you, you'll want to follow these steps to make sure you are picture perfect.

- Don't wear foundation with a sheen or dewiness to it. If you do, the strong light will make you look shiny, reflective, and oily in the photographs. Go as light as possible with your foundation; the light could make it visible. A lightweight foundation and a matte powder finish will photograph beautifully.

- Prep your skin well to make sure your foundation lasts throughout the ceremony and reception without needing a ton of touchups.

- Make sure your blush has a more matte finish. If it has too much shimmer, it will look too reflective in the photos.

- A crème blush is a great choice for this time of day. It will absorb into your skin and look more natural. Keep in mind that crème blush does not work well on oily skin, so stick with a powder blush.

- Because the light is so strong and can wash out your skin, highlighting and contouring is a must.

- Due to the midday lighting, if your eye makeup is too dark, your eyes will photograph like two dark holes. Your highlight shade is the most important shadow choice. Use a highlight with shimmer (not frost) to open up your eyes. The light-reflective particles in the shimmer will help prevent the "black hole effect."

- Make sure your midtone and/or contour shade has a matte finish—you never want to use three shades with shimmer, because your eyes will look too shiny in the photographs.

- If you want to wear eyeliner, keep it as close to the lash line as possible. If it is too thick, it could darken the lid more than you want, creating the dreaded "black hole effect."

- Long, beautiful eyelashes really help define your eyes without depending on heavy eyeliner (see page 136). False eyelashes would also be an excellent choice (see page 188).

- Because the sunlight grows stronger as the day advances, every makeup line becomes more visible on your face as midday approaches. Make sure to blend your foundation, blush, eyeshadow, and powder extremely well. At this time of day, there is no such thing as over-blending.

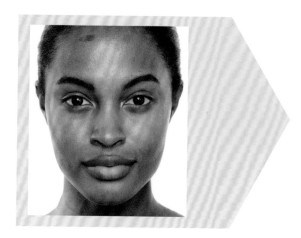

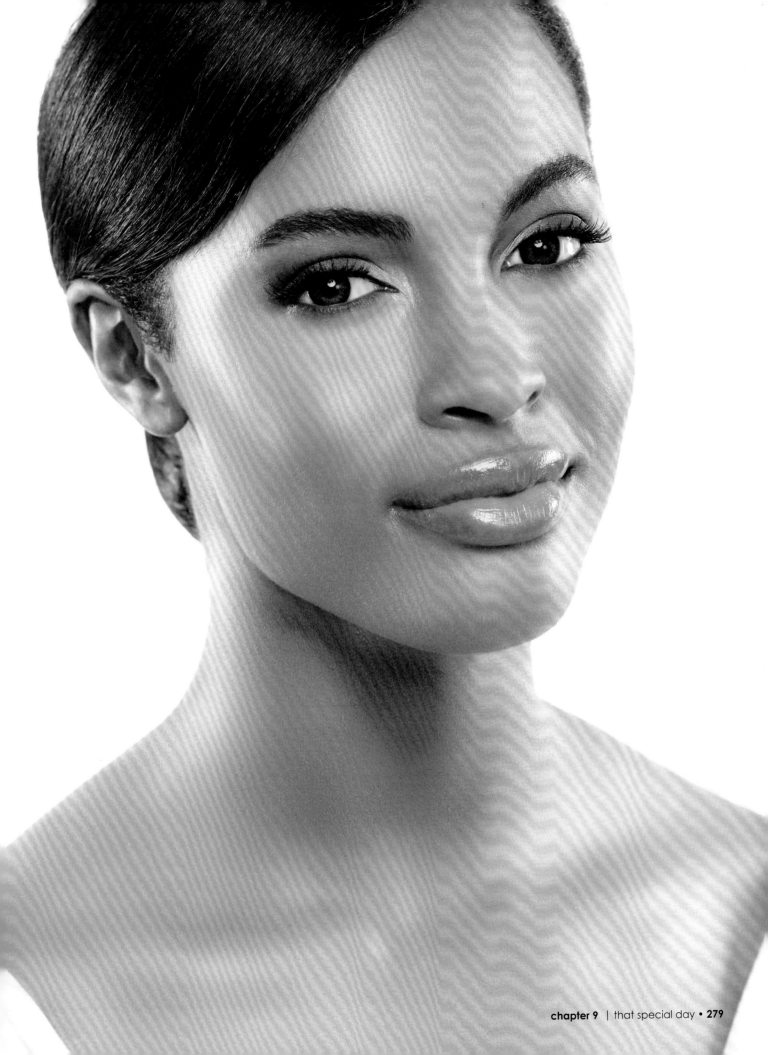

late afternoon bride

The golden light of late afternoon is the most beautiful light you can be photographed in. Late afternoon is when the sun is starting to set in the sky, creating a beautiful warm glow. Because the light will be so beautiful and forgiving, you can add a little more drama to your makeup look. You can wear more eyeshadow and have more shade options. This is hands down the photographer's and makeup artist's favorite time to photograph a bride.

- If your skin is less than perfect, late afternoon is a great time to get married. The light is softer and more forgiving, so you can use a little more foundation and concealer to cover your flaws, and your skin will still appear completely natural-looking in photographs. Don't forget to powder—remember that matte skin always photographs better than shiny skin.

- Make sure to prep you skin well so your foundation lasts throughout the ceremony and reception without a ton of touchups.

- As evening comes, your photographer will have to use a flash, so make sure you add color to your face. A flash shoots a bright burst of light in your face, which can make you appear washed out. Even if you do not normally wear blush, you need to wear at least a little color on your cheeks.

- Another way to prevent looking too pale or washed out in your photos is to contour your face and add a warm glow with bronzing powder (see pages 92 and 101).

- It's fine for your blush to have a little shimmert, because it will look beautiful in this light, though it is also fine if you want to use a matte shade.

- You can make richer color choices thanks to the lighting, so feel free to apply more dramatic eyeshadow shades.

- A shimmery (not frosted) eyeshadow will look beautiful because it photographs well in all lighting. Just make sure that your midtone and/or contour shade has a matte finish. You never want to use three shades with shimmer, because your eyes will look too shiny in photographs.

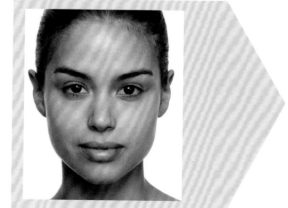

- Want to add a little more glamour? Try false eyelashes. This is the perfect time of day for this beauty trick, and eyelashes help define your eyes better than anything else you could do (see page 188). If you don't want to wear false eyelashes, just make sure to layer your mascara to get the most definition you can (see page 136).

- Late-afternoon brides get the green light to wear a richer lip color, too. The light allows you to wear richer colors without them showing up in photos as too intense.

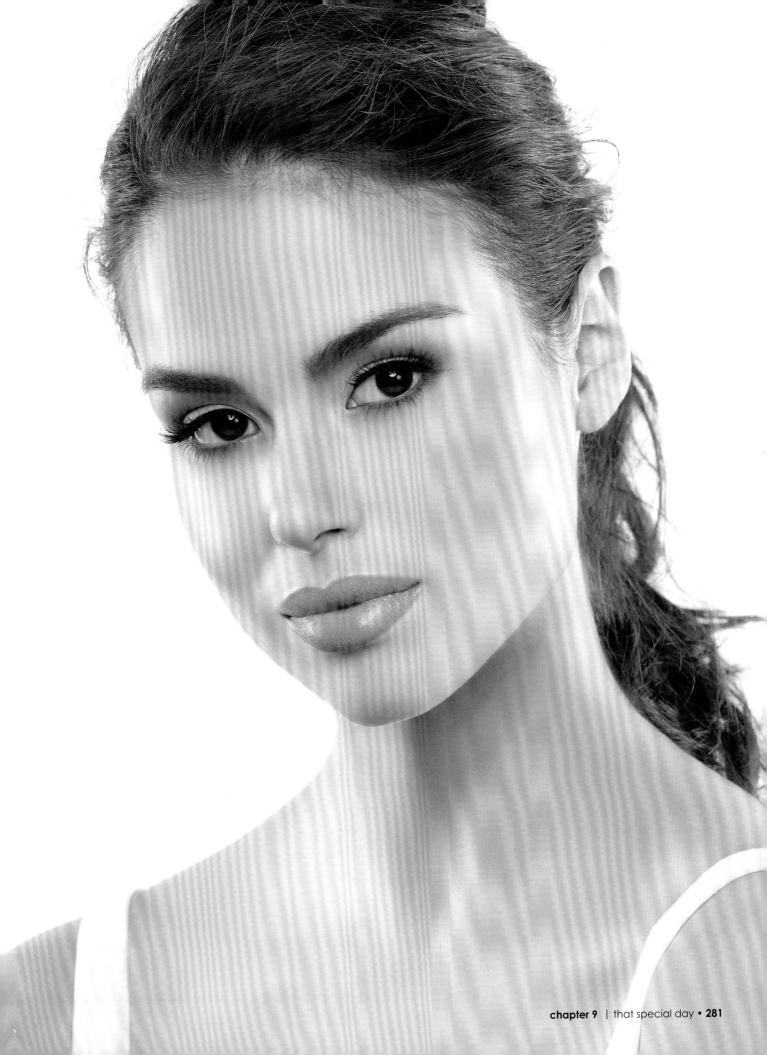

evening bride

If you love to glam it up, an evening wedding allows you to go for a more dramatic makeup look. You can play with color and wear more makeup at night than at any other time, and you will still photograph beautifully. This is the time of day for the bride who wants to be a glamour queen.

- If you have less than perfect skin, you can wear more foundation and powder at this time of day and still look natural.

- Make sure to prep your skin well so your foundation lasts throughout the ceremony and reception without needing a ton of touchups.

- Your photographs will be taken with a flash, so make sure to bronze generously to give your skin a glow. One thing that helps is sculpting your face, because it will add color so the flash will not wash your skin out, and it adds dimension. Dimension is important because the flash can also flatten everything out in a photograph (see pages 94 and 101).

- Everything should be more defined, from your lips to your eyes to your cheekbones, because all photos will be taken with a flash, which can wash you out. More defined does not mean darker. Even if you don't wear blush every day, you need at least a little color in your cheek for the flash. Give your lips a nice defined edge by lining them (see page 251).

- Even if you don't always wear brow color, you may need a little so your brows will show in the photos, especially if you're a natural blonde (see page 118).

- Shimmery eyeshadow will photograph well in the evening, but there should be absolutely no frosted shadows for this time of night (or any time for brides, in my opinion). Frosted eyeshadow looks too shiny in photographs, especially when a flash is used! A shimmery shadow always looks soft and pretty. Just make sure that at least one of your three shades of shadow is a matte. You never want all three shades to shimmer, because the eye will look too shiny in your photos.

- False eyelashes are a must for a nighttime wedding because they help define the eyes (see page 188). The more definition at your lash line, the better you will photograph. If you do not want to wear false eyelashes, layer your mascara (see page 136). This will also help to define them.

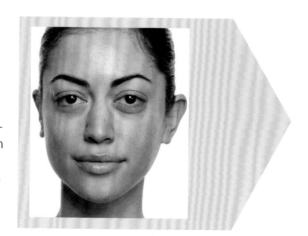

- If you want to wear a smoky eye, you're in luck. Evening is a perfect time for this eyeshadow application technique (see page 192). This look will photograph beautifully and look sophisticated. Just make sure to wear a soft lip color if you're wearing a smoky eye.

- Make sure you have lip color and powder on at all times. You never know when the camera will flash!

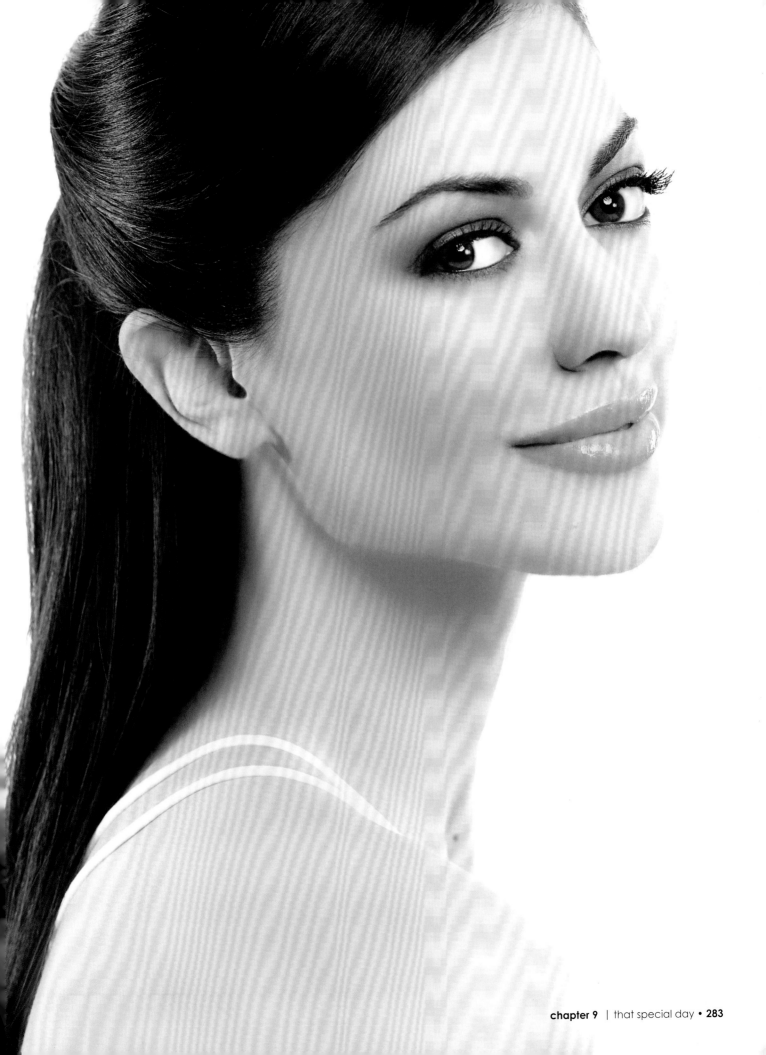

afterword

Whatever your goal is with makeup, I hope you reach it! That's true whether you just want to get better at applying your own makeup to increase your self-confidence or you want to go out and become the world's top makeup artist.

The joy I get from making people feel their most beautiful is immeasurable. I hope you find inspiration and continue to grow. There is inspiration all around you. You never know where it might come from: a movie, a friend, or an old picture of your grandmother. Embrace it all.

Whatever you do, don't lose sight of what makes you and each and every person you paint so special, their perceived flaws the things that make them different. We've learned to cover everything they might not want to see, but embrace the things that make them individuals and celebrate them.

Now that you have been armed with the knowledge about products and application, and knowledge is power, you have what you need to bring out your own or someone else's true beauty, their self-confidence. Just remember, no one can get good at anything without putting a lot of practice and hard work into it, so don't expect to be perfect from the start. Every day is a new chance to get it right and do it better than the day before. Practice, practice, practice.

Always remember, you cannot permanently harm anyone with makeup! It just washes off. So, don't be afraid to experiment. If you don't like it, wash it off and start over. One of the worst things we can do it get stuck in a rut and wear the same look for fifty years.

There are, of course, some hard and fast rules in makeup, which we have just learned, but never be afraid to venture out and try new things. You now know the basics and can use them to create anything you want. You can start to break the rules and be endlessly creative. I look forward to seeing great and wonderful things from you; I love seeing new talent and watching people grow. But most of all, I'm going to love seeing all of you walking around presenting your most confident self to the world. Embrace your own personal beauty—love who you are, today and every day!

infinitely yours—

about the author

Robert Jones did not necessarily start out on this career path. He showed promise as an artist as early as age 6 and was pushed—or maybe we should say encouraged—to pursue painting and drawing. He competed and won a scholarship to study at a prestigious art school at age 11. After seven long years of intense art training, he wanted more and decided to get more. From there, he attended a performing arts high school, where he majored in theatre. It is there that he first dabbled in makeup, applying painting principles to the face. Growing up with three sisters, he always had the opportunity to prove he was naturally gifted at working with hair. He was also able to put that talent to use in school performances. Upon graduating, his advisors expressed their belief that he should pursue his natural gifts. From there, he attended school and worked to get his license to do hair.

After years in a salon, he once again wanted more. With his life motto, "just jump and figure out how to make it work later," he got the opportunity to work with new models at an agency. From there, one thing led to another, and the rest is history. Now, after more than twenty-something years in the beauty industry, he has traveled the world working with so many amazing people.

His work has appeared in countless magazines, such as *Allure*, *Vogue*, *Marie Claire*, *InStyle*, *Life & Style*, *Glamour*, *Brides*, and *Elle*. He has worked with celebrities including Cindy Crawford, Claire Danes, Selena Gomez, Elaine Irwin, Eve Best (his favorite, he loves her), Sheryl Crow, Laura Linney, Natascha McElhone, Jennie Garth, Delta Burke, Diahann Carroll, and many others. He has worked with beauty and fashion clients such as Mary Kay, Almay, Olay, Avon, Nexxus, Clinique, Chanel, Prescriptives, Christian Dior, Neiman Marcus, Bergdorf Goodman, Saks Fifth Avenue, and Bloomingdale's, just to name a few.

Robert has a signature line of brushes and beauty tools available online at www.robertjonesbeauty.com and in stores soon. He also has an online makeup academy that can help anyone become the makeup expert he or she wishes to be at www.robertjonesbeautyacademy.com. This is his sixth book; he is also the author of the best-selling books *Makeup Makeovers*, *Makeup Makeovers: Weddings*, *Looking Younger*, *Makeup Makeovers: Beauty Bible*, and *Makeup Makeovers in 5, 10, 15, 20 Minutes*.

He has lived in Europe and New York, but now he has chosen to be back in Texas—with his other half, Chip, and fur babies, Gigi and Gretchen—as much as possible, especially because work keeps him in travel mode constantly.

index

liquids
blush, 28, 247
eyeliner, 23, 43, 133
eye shadow, 25
foundation, 13
pigment, 13
long-wearing lipstick, 30

m

mascara
curling mascara, 21
defining mascara, 21
layering, 136–139
lengthening mascara, 21
smudge prevention, 139
shelf life, 43
thickening mascara, 21
wands, 22
waterproof, 21
water-resistant, 21
matte eye shadow, 26
matte lipstick, 30
melasma, 78–79
midday bride, 278
moisturizer, 56
morning bride, 276
mousse foundation, 13

o

oil-free compact
concealer, 17
oily skin, 63
organic products, 42, 43

p

pencils
brow color, 19, 43, 118
concealer, 17
eyeliner, 23, 43, 132
eye shadow, 25
pigmented mineral
powder, 14–15
pomade brow color, 20,
43, 119
pony bristles, 32
pot concealer, 16
powders
blush, 27, 43, 245–246, 273
bronzer, 29, 43
brow color, 20, 119,
120–121
compact foundation, 14
eyeliner, 132
eye shadow, 25, 43
powder puffs, 41

powder (setting)
foundation and, 89
loose, 18
pressed, 18
shelf life, 43
primer, 57
prominent eyes, 174–179

r

rosacea, 81

s

sable bristles, 33
satin eye shadow, 26
sensitive skin, 63
sheer lipstick, 30
shelf life, 42–43
shimmer eye shadow, 26
shimmer lip finish, 31
skin
age and, 268
beards, 87–88
blemishes, 76–77
broken capillaries or
veins, 80
dark circles, 70–71
dark circles and
puffiness, 75
depth level, 62
facial masking, 83
hyperpigmentation,
78–79
hypopigmentation, 82
lip exfoliation, 57
melasma, 78–79
moisturizer, 56
primer, 57
rosacea, 81
scars, 84–85
tattoos, 85–86
types, 62–64
under-eye puffiness,
72–74
undertone, 61–62
vitiligo, 82
smoky eye, 192–197
sponges, 41
squirrel bristles, 32
stick concealers, 16
stick foundation, 13
storage, 42
synthetic bristles, 33

†

tattoos, 85–86
thickening mascara, 21
tinted moisturizer, 14
tube concealer, 16
tweezers, 41

v

vitiligo, 82

w

wand concealer, 16–17
waterproof mascara, 21
water-resistant mascara, 21
weddings
evening bride, 282–283
late afternoon bride,
280–281
midday bride, 278–279
morning bride, 276–277
wide-set eyes, 168–173